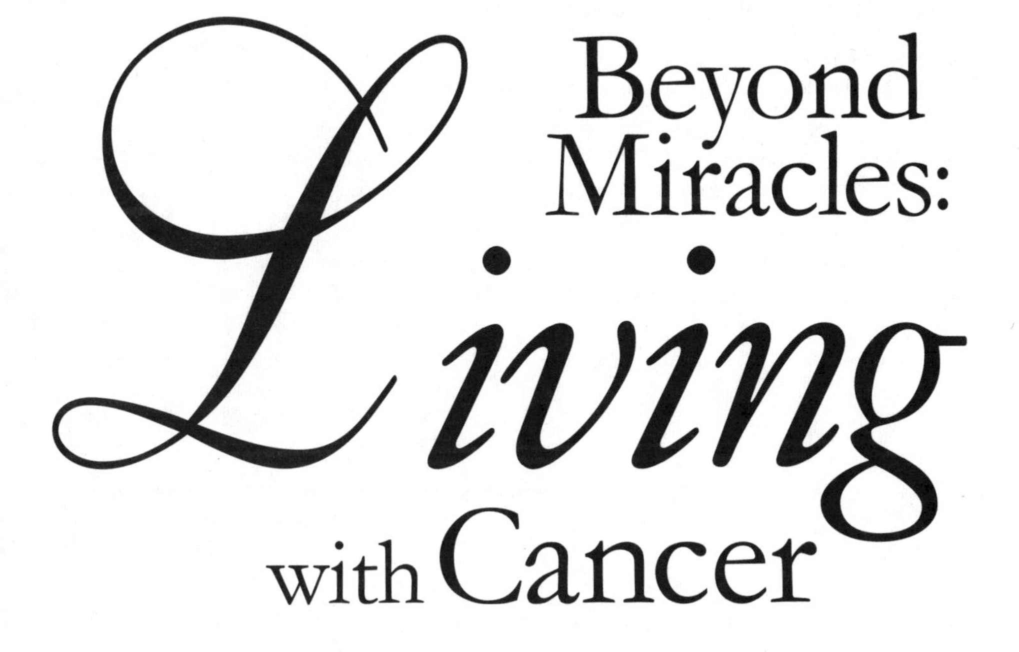

Beyond Miracles: Living with Cancer

Inspirational and Practical Advice for Patients and Their Families

STEPHEN P. HERSH, M.D.

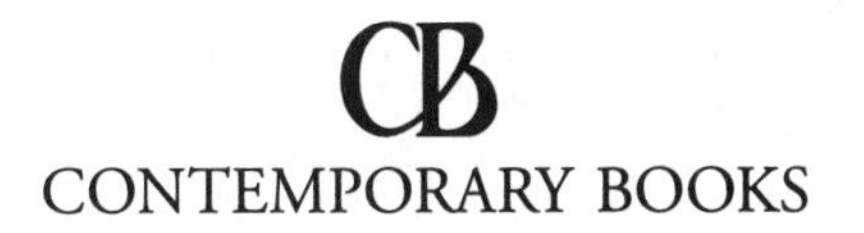

CONTEMPORARY BOOKS

Library of Congress Cataloging-in-Publication Data

Hersh, S. P. (Stephen P.)
Beyond miracles: living with cancer: inspirational and practical advice for patients and their families / Stephen P. Hersh.
p. cm.
ISBN 0-8092-3124-7
1. Cancer—Popular works. 1. Cancer—Psychological aspects.
I. Title.
RC263.H47 1997
362.1'96994—dc21 97-19628
CIP

Cover design by Monica Baziuk
Interior design and production by Susan H. Hartman

Published by Contemporary Books
An imprint of NTC/Contemporary Publishing Company
4255 West Touhy Avenue, Lincolnwood (Chicago), Illinois 60646-1975 U.S.A.

Printed in the United States of America
International Standard Book Number: 0-8092-3124-7
18 17 16 15 14 13 12 11 10 9 8 7 6 5 4 3 2 1

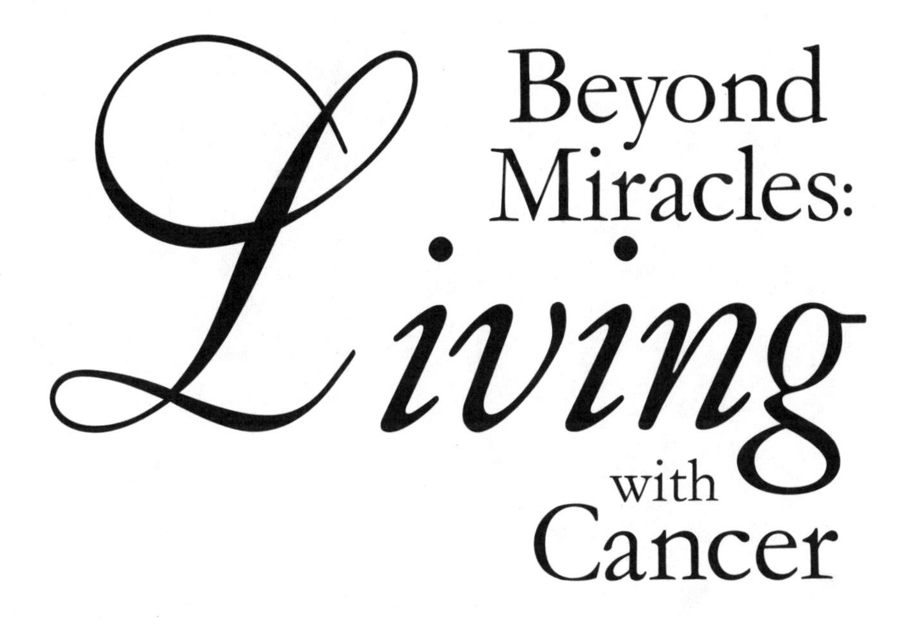

Beyond Miracles: Living with Cancer

To Joseph H. Hersh, M.D., F.A.C.S., and Lillian B. Hersh

Contents

"We are responsible just as much as doctors.
A person has to stop seeing himself or herself as
merely a patient and start participating
in the healing process."

D.S.—A veteran of cancer wars

Foreword

AS A TWENTY-FIVE-YEAR CANCER SURVIVOR and through my years with the National Coalition for Cancer Survivorship (NCCS), I have been fortunate to know many health care professionals who are dedicated to improving the quality of life for people living with cancer. Dr. Stephen Hersh is such a person.

Through his affiliation with NCCS and in a clinical practice devoted to helping people adjust to life following cancer, he demonstrates daily his belief in our guiding principle that *from the time of discovery and for the balance of life, an individual diagnosed with cancer is a survivor.* Our NCCS mission is to ensure that all cancer survivors (and their family, friends, and loved ones) are empowered with information that will help them live a better quality of life. Every page of this book reflects that goal.

With *Beyond Miracles* Dr. Hersh has given the cancer community an uncommon publication. His great sensitivity to both the biomedical and psychological needs of cancer survivors is too often lacking in standard medical practice. It is that quality combined with his distinctive passion for helping people and his considerable knowledge that makes this book as good as it is.

If you read it for specific details on a discrete topic, it can give you the necessary guidance on that subject. It is a book you can return to again and again to confirm a decision or to inspire some act of taking charge of your life as you deal with this fearful diagnosis. To get a comprehensive overview of what dealing with cancer is all about, along with practical tips on how to get through the most difficult times, this book can be read cover to cover.

Either way, you will get to know Steve Hersh as I have—as a caring, thoughtful, and compassionate person who exemplifies the kind of physician everyone with a cancer diagnosis should know. This book is no substitute for a trusted physician in your hometown, but Steve Hersh's insights in *Beyond Miracles* can inspire you to promote an even better relationship with your own doctor.

By learning from what he knows and has so eloquently written here, you can become a better-educated patient, a more effective communicator with your health care team, family members, friends, and coworkers. And you can turn to the book as a companion resource to get you through difficult or lonely moments during your treatment and recovery when communication with others is difficult.

Steve Hersh is a tireless supporter of our cancer community program as a speaker and participant. In addition, through his nonprofit Medical Illness Counseling Center he offers free seminars on a range of coping issues and cancer for anyone who wants to attend. Steve has learned from cancer survivors, and they trust him as they deal with their most feared experiences. When he is invited to a local support group meeting, he comes as both good listener and effective teacher. He does this in much the same way he counsels his private patients and in the way he presents difficult-to-read information in this book—with calm and understanding, offering both support and direction.

The desire to clone his manner of working with his patients is more than appealing. It is a sorely needed antidote to the cash-and-carry nature of today's cost-driven marketplace in which most of us now receive cancer care. (Other physicians who read this book could themselves provide a tremendous service to their communities by emulating Steve's participatory style and program.)

Beyond Miracles imparts a lot of truths, some of them hard to think about, much less accept. While you will learn in these pages that the medical profession can be a source of support and strength, you will also learn that the information you sometimes receive even from well-intentioned professionals can be misleading. You will learn how to react to these imperfections and to seek out those people who will take the time and make the effort to assist you in more than technical ways.

You will come to understand through this book how important your own outlook is as you move through your treatment, healing, and recovery process. But unlike some other popular self-help books, you will not be left with the sense of guilt that it is somehow your fault if your recovery is less than complete. Cancer, after all, is not a diagnosis emanating from your imagination but a real biological illness needing interventions at all levels of existence: the body, mind, and spirit.

This is a straightforward, fine book about dealing with the dreaded diagnosis of cancer. It is not a feel-good book, but it is a hopeful book—lacking platitudes but imparting the wisdom of a seasoned and well-respected physician. Understand what Steve Hersh has to say about coping with cancer, and his honest and direct guidance can help you build realistic optimism. Most important, the wisdom is here on how to live each day . . . beyond miracles.

—**Ellen L. Stovall,** *Executive Director,*
National Coalition for Cancer Survivorship
Member, National Cancer Advisory Board
of the National Institutes of Health (NIH)

Acknowledgments

FROM THE TIME I first began to think seriously about this book, I have benefited from the good humor, guidance, and editorial advice of a special friend, Norman Sherman. He suggested I write it, attended, in good health, my seminars for cancer patients to listen to the message I was conveying, helped me outline the book, and finally edited every chapter. Most of all he was a surrogate reader, making me explain the professional jargon my medical and scientific colleagues and I use in terms he understood, making me control my passion for overexplaining, lightening up the density of my prose, asking of me some of the questions that I suggest in this book you ask of your own doctors. This is my book, but it would have been much different without him.

Many friends in the health professions have advised me, informed me, guided me, and ultimately read what I have written. They include E. Fuller Torrey, M.D., and Professor Benjamin F. Hammond. Oncologists who checked me for accuracy on medical matters include Colonel Yvonne Andejeski and Allen Mondzac, M.D.; Vincent Devita, M.D., and Phil Pizzo, M.D., encouraged my interests on behalf of cancer patients beginning in the 1970s. Arthur S. Levine, M.D., offered me my original opportunity to consult and teach at the National Cancer Institute (NCI). Bertram Brown, M.D., supported my early involvement there and has been a caring mentor and close friend for more than twenty-five years.

I need to acknowledge especially the influence of Lucy R. Waletzky, M.D., my former colleague at the Medical Illness Counseling Center, who encouraged me in an openness and sensitivity to nontraditional approaches to helping patients. Ellen Stovall, who has graciously written the foreword, has by her example and commitment to cancer survivors been immensely inspirational in helping me understand the feelings and needs of cancer patients.

From the beginning, Jane Dystel has been more than an agent; she has been a wise guide and adviser throughout the development and writing of this book. Ginny Sherman has applied her copyediting and sense of literary style to the book as well. Ultimately, Susan Schwartz joined them as the person at Contemporary Books who took us from manuscript to finished book with valuable advice.

My wife, Jean, who has always been there for me in good times and bad, has provided the emotional support anyone needs in writing a book and a keen critical eye as well. She has helped me focus on this project, tolerating, if not always encouraging, the time stolen from family to be spent on the book.

I have dedicated this book to my father and mother, but that hardly captures the depth of my appreciation for their influence on my life and work. I learned early on from my father that there was joy in helping those who had health problems, in being a healer. And I learned, from his example, that you had to start with an affection for people and concern for their well-being. His passion was caring for others, and I served an apprenticeship of learning by accompanying him on hospital visits on cold winter days, on dark nights beyond my bedtime even as early as my tenth year. Weekends and holidays meant nothing to him, and I often tagged along as he dashed off to minister to the many surgical patients in his practice.

He was, and still is, a confident physician, but a gentle one, and simply always available to those in need. He has a ferocious dedication to honesty, intellectual integrity, and a never-ending passion for learning. I like to think I have been a good son, as well as a good physician, who has tried to follow his example.

My mother, a talented early female graduate of the Juilliard School of Music, put aside her career ambitions because she shared that sense of caring for those in need, an important part of her own family's dedication for decades before. It was a difficult choice of the mind, but an easy one of the heart. My father became for her more than husband and father of her children. He was a doctor in private practice, but a public servant in its truest meaning, and her admiration and respect and love for him drew her into his professional life whenever he needed her—office manager for years at a time, an assistant helping his nursing staff occasionally, and always, always a support.

Even today, as they approach ninety, he is still passionately learning; she, surrounded by the music she loves, remains a stalwart at his side. They are a wonderful couple. This book is, I hope, an extension of their lives.

Introduction: Listen, Learn, and Live

EVERY OTHER MONTH, as a physician whose specialty for the last twenty-five years has been a combination of behavioral medicine and psychiatry, I host a free discussion session for men and women who are suffering from a much-feared chronic disease called *cancer.* Some people come alone; more often they come with family members or a close friend. They come to me referred by their own doctors or attracted by newspaper accounts of what I am doing, but most often they show up simply because another person with a serious illness has told them about our meetings and the lessons they have learned that make their lives a little better.

Ultimately they come because the health care system has failed them—not in diagnosis or surgery or chemotherapy or radiation; they've frequently had plenty of that, and those services are generally quite good. The failure is something else. It is that our health care system does not listen to patients, especially concerning their fears. Nor does that system educate them about how to deal with their cancers, how to take back control of their lives, how to participate in their own healing.

Yet that participation is a vital part of any recovery plan. I cannot emphasize that enough. It is *the* essential first step toward doing well and feeling better. If you are passive and simply take what you get, what you get may not be what you need. Speak up. Ask questions. Make sure you understand. Ask again. Make decisions; don't just accept what others, no matter how professional, order.

Some people resist the move toward assuming such responsibility. Among them are those who wait, and hope, for a miracle. Miracles may occur. By definition they are exceedingly rare. (Between 1958 and 1984, more than two million people went to Lourdes on official pilgrimages. Of that number, sixty-four were recognized by the Catholic Church as having received miraculous cures. Of those sixty-four recorded by the Lourdes Medical Bureau, only four had cancer.)

Documented cases of unexplained remissions, even occasional complete disappearances, of a cancer do exist. Prayers for such events do provide solace to some people. But waiting for a miracle, even with lots of prayer, is a passive approach. A person who focuses only on prayer and miracles is betting against a stacked deck of cards.

I try to take my audience and my patients beyond miracles to an approach I know is more useful to them—striving to control their own lives and their own futures. I encourage, even excite, them to an emancipating struggle that lifts them out of the waiting game, its debilitating inactivity and passive acceptance of whatever the doctor orders.

Our American medical system, for all its excellence, too often leaves people feeling like victims—incapable of doing anything for themselves. I don't accept that condition, and neither should a person ill with even the most devastating disease. That is terribly wrong, particularly when the opportunity to do things differently is basic, inexpensive, human, neither technological nor intrusive.

In our meetings I don't diagnose anything; I don't prescribe any drugs. I just talk to those who have joined me about what I know about the human body, cancer, stress management, communication. I explain to them how much of their suffering can be avoided, that a vast amount of the physical and emotional misery that occurs in cancer patients, and by association also for their families, is unnecessary. And then I listen. The illnesses embodied in front of me are many and varied; what I hear, however, is almost a single voice. Yours could probably be added to the chorus.

Here's what I am told and know with certainty. Our current system focuses on *fixing*. Our culture demands *cures*. When they don't come easily or immediately, people often fall into anger, then depression, and are inclined to become passive—waiting for someone else or some miracle to make things right. This approach ignores important biological realities, including the wondrous capacities the human body has to care for, balance, and heal itself.

What we need as individuals and families is healing while scientists search for cures. Please understand this: Healing is different from being fixed or cured. Healing demands working with your body, encouraging its capacity for adjustment. Healing is impaired when you are in the victim mode waiting to be "fixed." How to step out of that devastating embrace of victimization, enhance your healing capabilities, and embrace life forms the substance of this book.

Much of what I have to say—and I am going to repeat some lessons over and over as if we were just talking to one another—grows out of my years of studying and working on the interaction between mind and body. Although I constantly immerse myself in the study of the latest advances in the biologic and medical sciences, cancer patients themselves have been my best instructors. With clarity and immediacy they have taught me lessons I had previously understood only in the abstract. Their message is clear: your feelings, thoughts, personality, and behavior are as important as your physical condition in good health and particularly when you become ill. If you are to make the most of the rest of your life, you must believe that. I am merely the conduit for this bit of wisdom and advice. It comes from people, possibly like you, who have heard the frightening diagnosis of cancer and have participated in high-quality clinical treatment research studies. They have dealt with the diagnosis realistically, with courage and determination, and most important, they have engaged in activities to improve their lives and healing. Their stories—composites with names changed to protect their identities—appear at various places throughout the text.

For the last fourteen years I have directed a nonprofit clinic, caring for individuals and families for whom medical illness has become a dominating factor in life. Our behavioral medicine center consists of psychiatrists, clinical nurse specialists, nurses, physical therapists, social workers, psychologists, and a nutritionist working together, recognizing that all healing skills do not reside in a single profession. The sum of our learning and skills is greater than the parts. We have developed considerable expertise in helping people live with and survive cancer. We educate our patients to step out of their victim mode—a natural reaction to bad news, of course, but not a healthy one.

Through education and enhanced skills we can all function at higher levels, and this is clearly true of someone beset by illness. Quality of life is improved by dealing with your problem, not giving in to it. Functioning within the family, community, and workplace gets better when you are determined to take control of your life. Responses to treatment are enhanced. And, for some, meaningful life is prolonged.

I wish I could talk to you face to face. I wish you could come to one of our seminars, but since that is not likely, this book must take the place of our gatherings. People who do come often use the same words to describe them: warm, engaging, nonthreatening, informative and helpful, easily understood, wide-ranging, serving to reduce fears. You ought to do what people there do. They ask questions. They challenge anything they don't understand or accept. It is the dialogue that is important, and I urge you to read and challenge and think about what I say here. Write to me about your own experiences and thoughts. Just putting your feelings down is likely to help you, even if you never mail the letter—although I hope you will. To the extent this book can create a sense of dialogue, of communication between you and me, I will have been successful in encouraging the healing process.

A wise man once said, "We all can engage in healing, learn to listen to our bodies and the world around us. As we do so, healing occurs through helping ourselves and others gain an improved sense of well-being as well as an improved sense of control. Joyful moments become more available; involvement with others through love more possible; and life itself—no matter what its length—a celebration."

If you remember only that, I will be a happy physician and author, and you will no longer be a captive of the victim mentality. That is the beginning of healing. That is the first step on the path beyond miracles.

1 The Fountain of Life Within You

*C*ANCER IS a frightening and powerful word. When you're told you have it, your heart rate goes up instantly, your head feels light, you may even feel a wave of nausea. Why shouldn't you? It is what every one of us dreads to hear. It sounds, in your initial shock, like a death sentence—immediate, inevitable, immutable. Devastating thoughts flow from the natural fear associated in our minds with cancer. Each of us, in that horrendous moment, feels the loss of control over our bodies and destinies. We think our bodies are falling apart and letting us down and victimizing us. We don't know why this has happened, and we don't know what to do.

Certain reactions to the news are almost universal. Fear begins. A part of you insists the doctor must be in error; the lab tests wrong. First disbelief fills you. Then you feel you are a victim of more than just your body—that you have displeased some higher power or, Joblike, you are being tested. You may, if you are not religious, believe at least that you are a victim of bad luck or evil demons like pollution, food you have eaten, chronic family or emotional conflict, technology, or your workplace. Who knows? In desperation you believe there has got to be a reason, an explanation, a definable cause. Your common sense and judgment are blunted. You feel impelled to immediate action. You want to be made better *now*.

The Diagnosis Is Not a Death Sentence

But hold on a moment! It is not that simple. To begin with, it is a common mistake to think of cancer as a single disease. We should really refer to *cancers* or *the diseases called cancer*. Indeed, the American Cancer Society should be called the American *Cancers* Society. The word *cancer* represents many conditions, for which there is no single cause and no single outcome. There are many kinds of cancer, and you—and even your doctor in many cases—cannot expect to know the consequences of your particular diagnosis with absolute certainty.

So what do we know? Great strides have been made in our knowledge. Every day more is being learned. At the moment, we know that what the cancers have in common is the out-of-control growth of a particular family of cells (soft tissue or blood or lymph nodes, or bone, or muscle, or brain, for example). That growth unbalances the normal relationships and functioning of the body, an unbalancing that if unchecked eventually threatens the survival of the whole person. But the key phrase is *if unchecked*. Until the middle of this century—really just a few decades ago—few successful treatments were available. That is no longer true. Today we know ways to check most cancers, and we will know more tomorrow. *The diagnosis of cancer is not a death sentence.* Some people live even with metastatic cancers for years; some cancers simply disappear; many are cured or put into remission for years. You must believe this and not give in to panic, despair, isolation from others, and passivity. While denial and unrealistic expectations don't help, collapse is not a reasonable or helpful alternative. So let's see if we can present certain facts that should help you.

Most cancers, with modern treatment, are illnesses that challenge the extraordinary capacity we have to heal, placing extra burdens on our physical and emotional selves, demanding an increased vigilance, and presenting the real possibility of a shortened life span. What does that mean for you? It means that uncertainty is a constant part of your life. It means that a cancer may be cured but that you must live with the thought that the cancer may return or that the probability of the development of a new cancer has been increased by your chemotherapy and/or your radiation treatments. Or it may mean that after treatment you will have no evidence of cancer in your body—the familiar term you've heard to describe this is *remission*—but because of the kind or stage of cancer you had your physicians feel they cannot use the word *cure*.

When a cancer disappears or "melts away" for reasons we don't understand, it is called *spontaneous remission*. For a rare few, a religious experience or a pilgrimage to a holy place seems to bring remission through a miraculous cure. While the possibility of remission and miracles provides hope for some people, there is certainly no scientific explanation, no way to cause or anticipate those changes. Yet there is absolutely no doubt that with or without medical treatment such events have occurred and continue to occur. While spontaneous remissions are rare, they are known to occur with other illnesses besides cancers. Their existence in any disease simply challenges our current understanding of biological processes.

What Are Your Chances?

Duane, extraordinarily successful at forty-seven years of age, was a person of great vigor with little need for sleep. When he noticed a dramatic change in his energy level over a period of months, he told his wife, who had herself seen the same changes, that he was too busy to see a physician about the change. (Later he realized he hadn't wanted to think that there might be a problem that he himself couldn't solve.) Then he began to lose weight. When he continued to do nothing, his wife and his best friend arranged a dinner where the two of them confronted him. It worked. Duane went to his physician, who found a colon cancer that had already spread to his liver. Still feeling stunned and with tightness in his chest, Duane asked the consulting oncologist, "How long do I have?"

Maryanne's breast biopsy was positive for cancer. Aggressive chemotherapy began when tests showed that her breast cancer had spread to other parts of her body. The response was extraordinary—soon no evidence of tumor could be found. "I've beat it," she announced to her doctor. He shook his head and gently explained that cancer treatment was not a black-and-white thing. Dramatic positive response did not mean cure. Angrily, thinking he was announcing her death sentence, she demanded, "Well, what are *my chances?"*

If there is anything certain in cancer diagnosis, it is that everyone thinks or asks "What are my chances?" not once but many times. "Will I be cured?" "Will I survive?" "How long will I live?" People seek certainty when none exists. We all seem to prefer being told a specific time period by a doctor rather than the truth, which is "I don't know."

When someone—your doctor or someone on your medical team—tells you that you have six months, a year, or two years to live, he or she is just guessing. That guess is based on information developed from various studies, but it is just a guess. Studies depend on a sampling of identified cancers in people who have presented themselves for treatment and study. Scientists translate the results of these studies into probability curves, but generalizations drawn from probabilities do not apply to any particular individual.

The course of your illness may or may not be described by that statistical curve, because our studies are not based on everyone with a particular kind of cancer but only on those who have been part of a study. No physician can predict exactly where any patient will fall on a statistical curve. At best this approach supplies reference points for you and your doctor, allowing some planning and assisting in decision making.

To tell an individual how long he or she will live is both inappropriate and utter nonsense. Don't ask your doctors "How long have I got?" Or, if you must ask, take the answer with a large grain of salt. Don't accept declarations about your life span. There is absolutely no way any physician can know how long you will live. (Many patients have attended funerals of physicians who appeared healthy when they pronounced a short life expectancy for the patient.) Focus on the reality that you are alive. Be determined to live as long and as well as you can.

Must You Change Your Lifestyle?

The important thing to remember is that any chronic illness, including cancer, demands changes in lifestyle, changes in how you use your energies, your time, and other resources. *Cancer demands a reordering of priorities.* But believe me, that does not mean giving in or giving up hope.

In the early stages of expanding his plumbing business, Kevin was both furious and disbelieving when his doctor told him that the growth on

his vocal cord that made him hoarse was cancerous. Surgery and chemotherapy and radiation would be needed as treatments. My God, he thought, I don't even have enough time now for my kids. How am I going to fit in the treatments, too?

Cancer does mean using common sense aggressively, not casually. For instance, your treatments may suppress your immune functions, making you more vulnerable to contagious illnesses such as flu or viral and bacterial pneumonias. Since crowds are likely places to catch these illnesses, it is wise during periods of immunosuppression to avoid spending much time in close spaces with many people. You may end up watching videotapes at home rather than going out to crowded movie houses. You may want to avoid rush-hour bus or subway trips. You should avoid sharing cups or eating utensils with others.

Elena loved her work as a school nurse, her church volunteer commitment, and especially her role as mother to a child still at home and two older daughters who still came to her for advice. She made no time for exercise or recreation since her days were so crowded. When she noticed a really dark and crusty area on her heel, she did make time to see her family doctor and then at his insistence a dermatologist. The diagnosis was malignant melanoma, which would require immediate surgery and possibly other treatment. As she struggled with the fact of her illness, she thought, How can I make time? I already have so many commitments.

Both Elena and Kevin experience what confronts everyone when diagnosed with cancer: the need to alter thinking and behaviors. This need places on them the additional burden of very *normal* emotional reactions that include protest, resentment, anxiety, and perhaps even feelings of depression. What their initial distress expresses is feelings of being overwhelmed by the changes that the situation requires. Both Elena and Kevin need to direct their energies toward the new priorities presented by their cancer diagnoses and let go of their usual priorities and the behaviors that follow from those priorities. This harsh reality forces a new perspective from which their needs change to finding the best treatment available and improving self-care. After some struggle, this change will ideally be experienced by them as their choice *in the context of their circumstances*. Reinforcing ties to their closest family members and friends and participating as knowledgeable consumers in the treatments administered become additional priorities. Perhaps you find yourself confronted with challenges similar to those facing Elena and Kevin. Personal strength and discipline are required to cope with the changes in the use of your energies, time, and lifestyle.

Why You?

Even before you deal for very long with lifestyle and survival questions, you will feel compelled to ask why you got the disease. What causes cancer? What caused *your* cancer? With a cancer diagnosis, every one of us involved wants an answer, preferably in the form of an easily understandable explanation. No matter how old we are, we are like two-year-olds who relentlessly keep asking "Why?" We all learn by asking and listening. Unfortunately, there are no easy answers.

Our bodies aren't made that way. Each of us is a biological system, and virtually nothing about us can be totally explained by one action, event, or happening. Many variables determine the functioning and changes in our biological systems.

The human body is a magnificent creation composed of a highly complex pattern of specialized cells working together and communicating through chemical and electrical interactions. Our cells interact with each other and react to our external and internal environments in a wondrously ever-changing way. We are only at the beginning of knowledge about how the miracle of our bodies works.

There is another reason we cannot easily answer the "Why?" question. For some cancers we have ideas about significant influencing factors, but that is not the same as knowing the cause. Maybe this distinction is clearer in a nonmedical example. If you don't know much about cars, you might say that a foul-smelling liquid, gasoline, and some funny round things, tires, cause the car to move. You'd be wrong, of course. They are significant influencing factors, but they do not cause the car to move—the internal combustion engine connected to gears and crankshaft does.

The medical profession is, in some ways at some times, just like you in that automotive example. We can identify significant influencing factors, but we may not be able to identify the combined causes. We may think we know, but our hypothesis may be wrong. Even when we can objectively distinguish the various roles of tires and gasoline and the internal combustion engine, we may still be only on the edge of understanding. Medicine, however much we would hope otherwise, is both an evolving and an imprecise science; while cancer research has brought great advances, we still operate in gray areas of partial knowledge. What is important is that each of us—physician or patient—understand this and ask every question that may lead to a more complete answer in a specific case. For a doctor, that means a better chance to figure out what is happening; for the patient, that means a fighting chance to make the best, most informed decisions about treatment and self-care.

A Look at Some of the Cancers

Let me give you an example from our half-illuminated cancer world—the Hodgkin's form of lymphoma. We believe that the Epstein-Barr virus (EBV) may have something to do with Hodgkin's disease, and we also know that Epstein-Barr is the agent that causes mononucleosis. We don't have the foggiest idea why some people with the Epstein-Barr virus have no mono symptoms but show evidence in blood tests of having encountered the organism. Mono can be serious, but often it is just a passing misery for young people kidded by their peers for having the "kissing" disease.

Yet *some* people with Epstein-Barr *may*, years later, develop Hodgkin's disease. Why the Epstein-Barr virus may tilt the balance in the direction of some people becoming ill with a form of cancer while others simply become chronic hosts to the virus is not understood at this time. We believe Epstein-Barr is a significant influencing factor. We cannot yet say what the cause of Hodgkin's is. To use that automobile metaphor again, we don't know for certain if the Epstein-Barr virus is the internal combustion engine or the fuel or plays another essential role.

Looking further at the EBV-cancer connection, we are more certain of the connection with two other forms of cancer. The EBV infection is now considered the necessary initial event for the development of Burkitt's lymphoma in East African populations and nasopharyngeal cancer in Africa, China, and Southeast Asia. Even though EBV infections abound in the United States, nasopharyngeal cancer in particular is rare here while common in the geographic areas just listed. Yet many infected with EBV in those countries get neither form of cancer.

Geography and racial groups as they relate to cancer raise many questions and give few answers. Japan, for example, has very low rates of Hodgkin's disease, testicular cancer, Ewing's sarcoma, superficial spreading melanoma, chronic lymphocytic leukemia, and Wilms' tumor but very high rates of stomach cancer. Female Japanese immigrants to the United States have an incidence of endometrial carcinoma that is two times greater than that of Japanese women who do not emigrate. However, those who do come here have much lower risks of cervical cancer. (And, what, if anything, does geographic location have to do with the three known risk factors for endometrial cancer—obesity, absence of pregnancies, and polycystic ovaries?)

Native Americans, while suffering from significantly higher rates of diabetes than others in the United States, have much lower cancer rates than Caucasians. So what are the influencing factors: Environmental factors such as cleanliness or mineral content of water, exposure to heavy metals or coinfections with bacteria, fungi, viruses, or parasites such as malaria? Nutrition? Human genetics? Or a combination of all these factors? We just don't know.

Let's take a look at another illness. There are forms of cancer of the colon, or large bowel, that are known to run in families. Indeed, having two or more relatives with a history of bowel cancer is considered a significant risk factor for a form of cancer called *adenocarcinoma of the large bowel.* That tells us something, but certainly not who will get cancer and who will not.

A Glance at Genetics and Families

In recent years scientists have found faulty genes on several chromosomes that are associated with a predisposition to bowel cancer. That tells us more; not enough, however, to predict tomorrow's cancer patient. Soon a blood test will be available to identify these faulty genes—genes that may occur in at least one in two hundred people. If we can identify who has those faulty genes, can we know who will get cancer? Clearly not. Some with the faulty genes will get it, and some will not. Yet such a test would allow us to identify a group of people who should receive regular screening for bowel cancer. Such an effort is worth the cost, because early diagnosis alone followed by proper treatment can cure up to 90 percent of those who get bowel cancer.

There are other cancers that seem to run in families. Certain kidney cancers strike some families disproportionately, particularly those with many cysts in their kidneys. Many of you have heard of families in which the incidence of breast cancer has been high over generations. For all these cancers, genetics are an influencing factor.

The rare cancer family syndrome called Li-Fraumeni (LFS), after the two scientists who identified it, represents one of the most dramatic examples of cancer genetics in humans. This syndrome involves the *rare* occurrence of an inherited p53 tumor suppressor gene mutation. Members of Li-Fraumeni syndrome families have many often fatal tumors involving sarcomas, other solid tumors, brain tumors, breast cancer, leukemia, and lung and adrenocortical tumors.

Although important, sometimes even dramatic, as with the LFS, genetic background does *not* fully explain the expression of the disease; that is, why some members of such families develop cancer and respond poorly to treatment, others respond well, and others do not develop the disease at all. We in the medical profession do not have all the answers.

All we can really say is that environmental and genetic factors play joint roles in an individual's medical history. It is important, for example, to realize that we live in a close relationship with lots of different microorganisms in the forms of viruses, bacteria, and fungi. Most do not make us ill. Some may even be necessary for health.

The Environment

On the other hand, substances from the environment may be significant contributing factors to cancer. Among these are the various forms of coal tars. People can be exposed to them through occupational hazards. Historically the connection was noted between solid tumors in young boys who were chimney sweeps in England in the late nineteenth and early twentieth centuries. Today, of course, the most commonly known connection with coal tars and cancer involves ongoing use of any form of tobacco. That is particularly true with the development of cancer of the lip, tongue, mouth, bowel, and lung. Coal tars may also have an influence on the development of cancers of the bladder and breast. Radon is known to cause certain lung cancers. Benzene, a solvent chemical widely used and widely distributed in our air and water, is a proven causative agent in certain forms of leukemia. And, of course, most people are aware today of the role ultraviolet light plays in causing both localized skin cancers and malignant melanoma.

The fact that cancers can be associated with certain infectious agents, environmental hazards, or genetics represents the reality of our biological world. Consider for a moment illnesses that are known to be caused by infectious agents such as typhoid or tuberculosis or diphtheria. A wide range of factors determines how an infected individual's body handles the infection. The infectious agent in combination with the degree of exposure to it, the preexisting general health of the person, and genetic and environmental factors determines outcomes that range from having little or no overt clinical illness to becoming overwhelmed by the organism very quickly and dying. Based on the same principles, our responses as individuals to the cancers vary.

Thus each of us is unique, even with an illness such as cancer. No doctor, no study, can tell you what your particular responses will be. You can be presented with possibilities and probabilities. It is your responsibility to pursue to your utmost your own healing, making use of what the medical profession has to offer. Therein lies your hope, your future.

2 Clinic and Hospital Experiences: Getting Beyond Survival to Hope

ONE ELOQUENT SURVIVOR of cancer, Reynolds Price, wrote in his superb book *A Whole New Life* about his experience with the medical profession, hospitals, and the entire health care system. At one point he wonders whether patients should be able to demand a kind of consumer warning about the character of physicians they may encounter. In particular, he suggests warning labels on the offices of those he calls "flawed practitioners." He has written his own: "Expert technician. Expect no more. The quality of your life and death are your concern."

You'd do well to heed Professor Price's advice. Learning how to work with doctors, nurses, and other medical staff is vital to your success in dealing with your illness. Trust in those you depend on is, of course, important, and inevitably you must depend on many people—on their knowledge, experience, integrity, and compassion. Your trust, however, must be supported by what you actually experience. People do become victims of medical practitioners and the medical care system as well as of their illness. To avoid that victimization, and it is certainly something to be avoided, you need to understand the strengths of the people you will see *and* their limitations, as well as how the system works. Today, in the face of managed health care driven by the motives of for-profit business, this understanding is more critical than ever.

You need to look at medical personnel—doctors, nurses, aides—with a clear view, evaluating them on the quality of their actions and statements. And you need to understand hospitals, procedures, and tests. You need to develop skills in dealing with the people you depend on so you can make the best of your situation. At a time when you want to look inward, you must monitor everything that is going on around you. Only then can you find ways of making the system work well for you. Only then can you hope to avoid becoming, or remaining, its victim.

How to Work with Doctors

Reynolds Price had another special insight in his book. He said, "And surely a doctor should be expected to share . . . the skills of human sympathy . . . letting another creature know that his or her concern is honored and valued." Unfortunately, not all doctors do.

So, you must start with a good look at the physicians in your life. If you think your doctor is all-powerful and infallible, you begin with a serious misconception. (Some of my colleagues do suffer from that distorted view of themselves, but that is no reason for you to accept it.) Doctors of medicine are just people. This simple reality often gets lost or submerged when you are faced with a serious illness. Overwhelmed by the anxiety that accompanies your condition, you easily become a supplicant at a "temple of healing," making your doctor more than he or she is, almost like some Greek god or powerful priestess of old. A supplicant begs for help and accepts what is given. That is unhealthy for both you and any doctor honored as high priest.

Understanding Physicians

Physicians, I repeat, are just people. We know some things you don't. We have special knowledge of human anatomy and physiology in health and in disease. We have been trained to do special, sometimes almost mysterious, things. Yet we face the same life challenges, suffer the same moods that you do—perhaps even the same fears. We may have a fulfilling life outside of work, or we may not. We may have our own health problems. However much money we make, we may still have intense economic pressures or unraveling personal relationships.

Most of us care deeply about what we do and how we do it. But since we are people, just like plumbers, teachers, and lawyers, we have among us our own array of saints, sinners, heroes, mediocre people, and just plain jerks. A person of good common sense once noted that 50 percent of the doctors you meet finished in the bottom half of their class and never sought to rise above that level.

As physicians, if we suffer, we should suffer in silence as far as our patients are concerned. By tradition, we are supposed to reveal to patients little or nothing of our nonprofessional selves. That is proper. You don't go to a doctor to hear his or her problems. No doctor should open up and tell everything to everybody. For the patient, a physician ideally presents a professional demeanor: a self-assured, commanding, focused, hopefully caring presence.

We are trained over an extended period—often ten years of medical school, residency, specialty fellowships, and certification in the mysteries of the human body, its functions in health and especially in illness. Those are years of extraordinary intensity and self-absorption. There is little time and no reward for self-doubt as we struggle with molecules, genetics, cellular and subcellular systems, anatomy and physiology, disability, illness, public health, birth, growth and development, surgery, medications, and other aspects of the healing arts.

Many of us may become quite like bodybuilders: overfocused and often overdeveloped in certain ways. Doctors pay the price of imbalance because of little formal training in relating to and communicating with people. Beyond mirroring the behavior we observed of our residents and faculty supervisors, we receive little or no instruction in handling or managing people when they are either in normal health or distressed. As a result, many of us have not made enough time to develop interpersonal skills, capacities for listening to or respecting the thoughts and feelings of others.

Even the best of us, chronically living with more work than we can efficiently handle, do not always treat individuals, situations, or ourselves as well as we should. We too get grumpy, irritable, fatigued. We too will deny fatigue is impairing our judgment. We too have trouble saying "No, we cannot handle more." We too struggle with honesty. We too make mistakes.

None of this is an apology; nor is it meant to excuse the poor physician. It is meant to help you be realistic about us. Through such understanding you, I hope, will be encouraged not to be in awe of us (or, on the other hand, to fear us). Respect is enough to make the relationship work at its maximum in your behalf. But respect does not mean unquestioning acceptance of everything you are told.

(Ironically, when doctors become ill, they are frequently lousy patients, demanding, querulous, challenging, only partially compliant. Possibly because of our experiences, we are not inclined to trust fully other doctors, nurses, or the medical system.)

Your body is *your* body; its illness is *your* illness; your life is *your* life. We have the knowledge and skills to help with all three—body, illness, life—but we do our best, and you heal best, when you see our work as a collaboration between us. So, no matter how much we care, *you must care more*; you must be your own prime and forceful advocate.

The Role of Your Family Physician

If you are fortunate enough to have a primary-care physician (family doctor, general practitioner, pediatrician, or internist) with whom you have had a good, trusting relationship, don't give it up. All too often, once a person is diagnosed with cancer, he or she is swept into the world of specialists. That may be inevitable and necessary, but it does not mean that an important, useful, and understanding relationship with your regular doctor should end. In fact, the primary-care physician should be your sounding board to whom the specialist reports and with whom you should discuss any recommendations.

Specialists too frequently, almost routinely, leave your primary-care physician out of the communication and treatment loop if you permit it. And that almost inevitably puts you at a disadvantage as an isolated patient. Your family doctor has known you in sickness and in health in a kind of medical marriage. Your primary-care family physician should be a vital and continuing general advocate for your physical health, for your understanding of recommendations, and often for your quality of life.

Hence you should let your primary-care physician continue to help you monitor all aspects of your health, interpret findings for you when needed, reassure you, and assist you in advocating for yourself in the medical system. In fact, there are some cancer treatments that can just as well be administered by your family doctor, working in consultation with an oncologist, thus often saving you time and money. Some cancers are currently treated in highly standardized ways, almost like recipes in a cookbook. The role of the family doctor under these conditions is important to understand and is particularly important and useful for those who live far away from major cancer treatment centers.

What Is an Oncologist?

The basic training of all doctors is largely the same during the first three years of medical school. Only after that does it begin to change, as beginning physicians move toward family practice, pediatrics, internal medicine, surgery, or some other specialty. Doctors who focus, usually after training in internal medicine or pediatrics, on the different forms of cancer and blood diseases are the oncologists and hematologists. They study how cancer and blood diseases affect and disrupt the body's normal functions and the different ways of treating these conditions—radiation, chemotherapy, surgery, immunotherapy. An oncologist's specialty—what sets that particular doctor apart from others—is the special knowledge of what appropriate and available treatments may help the body fight off or control the disease and how to use those treatments while supporting the body's functions.

Oncologists must master immense amounts of technical information, beginning with lab tests of body fluids, x-rays, CAT scans, MRIs, medications and their toxicities. While tracking the cancer's response to treatment, an oncologist must monitor the patient's salt and acid-base balance, hydration and nutrition, immune system functioning, liver and kidney functioning, pain, and other discomforts and must check for infections. Some oncologists specialize in particular forms of cancer, such as breast cancer, sarcomas, or brain tumors; most are generalists. Some may focus on particular treatment approaches: radiation therapy, surgical oncology, or chemotherapy.

There are an estimated thirteen thousand such specialists in the entire United States. Yet more than ten million people are living with some form of diagnosed cancer, either in active treatment or having completed treatment. One million new cancers are diagnosed each year. Some oncologists have done more than taken special training in treating cancer; they have sought certification by the American Board of Hematology and Oncology. With this certification the community, other doctors, and patients have reassurance that an individual's training and mastery of the subject are at the highest level recognized by others who specialize in the field. It is comforting to know that your doctor has attained this level of knowledge.

Cancer Doctors and Compassion

What board certification doesn't guarantee is that the doctor has the compassionate skills of caring, an openness to your being a member of the treatment team, and a good bedside manner. Nor does it guarantee that he or she will work with you as a whole person rather than as a person with an interesting disease. (Both traditions exist in Western medicine. When Sir William Osler held the chair of medicine at Oxford University, he was described as charming to patients and students alike. His successor, Sir Archibald Garrod, focused on the biochemical individuality of humans; he was described as detached and interested chiefly in his patients' urine.) Whether your doctor is good at communicating or not, whether certification is there or not, you need always to ask questions and not stop asking them until your questions have elicited answers that make sense to you. Whatever your kind or level of education, a knowledgeable physician interested in you can explain anything you need to know in terms you can understand.

If you are lucky, your oncologist will instinctively have the human skills that are so vital to a successful treatment. Unfortunately, too often the need to master other details precludes training in such communication and psychological skills. Very few doctors are tuned in to the emotional states of their patients or even to the inevitable irritability and fatigue in all those who are receiving treatment or suffer from chronic pain. The reason is quite simple. Not many doctors have been patients themselves; lacking that, their insights and empathy are limited.

Indeed, knowing how to diagnose or treat cancer brilliantly does not necessarily include any true sense of how patients feel and think or how the illness of cancer affects the lives of the patients and their families. It is odd, but true, that medical specialists such as oncologists may be even less likely than primary-care physicians to be supportive and empathetic to patients and their families. A very gifted oncologist once said to me, "I don't know nor do I think about what my patients' lives are like between appointments." In part this is a reaction to the stress of their work: 100 percent of their patients have complicated, severe illnesses. At most, only 40 percent of a primary-care physician's patients are so ill. Distancing oneself from patients and family serves to protect the oncologist's emotions, freeing him or her to focus on the technical aspects of care.

Working with Your Cancer Doctors

From the time of meeting the new patient, the oncologist will tend to charge ahead aggressively, focusing on the cancer, lab tests, other studies, and treatments. Rarely will he or she look at you and ask how you are reacting to all of this emotional as well as physical turmoil, whether things are happening too fast, whether you have any questions about what is being done to your body, how much you want to have explained, or how much you understand.

The first thing for you to do after a diagnosis of cancer is to be sure that your doctor has obtained an independent second opinion based on your history, physical examination, and data from the test results and pathology reports. If not, you should seek one yourself. That does not indicate distrust of your doctor, even if he or she is a certified oncologist, but simply advocacy for yourself. No competent physician will be hurt or affronted by such a request. With such a serious diagnosis, the doctor should applaud your request and even help set up such a consultation.

We doctors, as I have said over and over again, are people who have been well trained, but who, like everyone else, make errors from time to time. Slides from tissue samples have been known to be mixed up. A slide can be misinterpreted. You have undoubtedly read of such errors or heard of them in your own community. Beyond error, honest differences of opinion can occur in a diagnosis.

Alicia, twenty-five years old, cut her leg while shaving. A dark mole was in the area of the cut. It became inflamed. Her husband, an oncologist in training, panicked, thinking she had, by the trauma, started the injured mole on a process of change into a melanoma. A dermatology consultant agreed and performed a wide, deep incision biopsy. The first pathology diagnosis: early invasive melanoma. Further disfiguring leg surgery was recommended to be followed by chemotherapy. Fortunately, her slides were sent to several experts around the country before any additional treatments were begun. Their conclusion: cellular changes consistent with injury and no melanoma!

Since we cannot deny that human errors are possible, although not frequent, you must protect yourself as well as you can by reducing the probability of such errors before you start treatment. A second opinion is a good way to start. Even being sure the problem is cancer is not sufficient. When the diagnosis is made correctly as cancer, an accurate determination of the cell type is a very important factor influencing the treatments used.

Differences exist not only on whether there is cancer and what type of cancer it is but, equally important, on how advanced it is. All of this simply underlines what you need most—confidence that the doctor knows with some precision what is going on. You need reassurance that the physicians working with you have no doubt about what cancer you have, how aggressive and advanced it has become, and what can be done to treat it. You want to determine that you can hopefully and realistically do well with the known treatments.

And that may sometimes come only with a third opinion. Seeking another opinion when there is no doubt, no difference of opinion, no confusion may be a fatal form of denial—delaying treatment after it should have begun. But when legitimate medical differences exist, it is appropriate to look for a third opinion from a world-class expert in your form of cancer. Such opinions can often be provided responsibly without your having to travel to see that expert. Your age, sex, medical history, slides, and lab and other test data can be transmitted easily to those consultants.

Choosing Your Cancer Doctor

In choosing the specialist you work with (oncologic surgeon, medical oncologist, or radiation oncologist), there are several factors that you need to focus on. The first, of course, is the person's background, which you can learn ahead of time. This includes the individual's experience in the field (how long and how many cancers of your type he or she has seen) and whether he or she is working with other individuals who have similar or greater experience. The second has to do with management style. Is the physician or the clinic or office run in a way that you feel allows you to gather information, ask questions, and participate in your own care in ways that work for you? Other patients may give you some insight into this area, but you may have to visit the office yourself.

Information gathering, questioning, and participation vary greatly from one person to the next. There are certainly many individuals who would rather have minimal information, believing deeply, if not totally, in their doctor's skill and knowledge. But for others—for most of you, I hope—it is very important that the doctor come across as an individual who conveys a feeling of your importance and demonstrates willingness to listen to you. This will be discussed further in the section on communication.

Many people choose a physician specialist with less care than when they buy a refrigerator or a car or get the house painted. People usually check around, comparison-shop, read magazines with product ratings, go to a library. Yet with cancer treatment you are dealing not with some inanimate object but with your quality of life—and life itself. Make at least the same kind of careful analysis about your medical support as you would about your car.

Find out what you can about your doctor. Be a consumer activist for yourself. Do more than simply accept the referral given to you by another physician. Physicians, just like everyone else, often refer patients to colleagues working in the same system or to acquaintances, friends, or just golfing partners. Gather information about training and years in practice of the oncologist to whom you are referred. Feel free to check the library in your community, which probably has a directory of certified medical specialists describing their backgrounds. You may even find the names of specialists who look more attractive to you. If possible, discuss what you have learned with your primary-care doctor to obtain his or her views. (See Appendix E for resources.)

As they begin their practices, physicians, no matter how brilliant and accomplished, do not have the hands-on experience you ideally want. If, however, a younger physician makes you feel comfortable, work with him or her. What you give up in experience may be compensated for by mutual trust and ease of communication.

But again, remember that a physician, like any professional or anyone plying a trade, does grow and develop with experience. Add such professional experience with a consultation if it is not readily available from one physician. For your second, backup opinion, you should seek someone with ten years or more of experience beyond postspecialty training. That guarantees that you will have the advantage of different perspectives, consideration of different treatments and supportive care. The breadth of experience can and often does make a significant difference in your care.

Once you have established your oncologist's credentials, pay attention to how the physician communicates with you and how his or her office works. There are brilliant physicians who communicate poorly. But they may have a team of receptionists, nurses, and technicians who make up for their personal lack of skills. Do not stick with a treatment situation, no matter what the credentials of the physician, if you are not generally treated with directness and respect and if your need to participate in the treatment process is significantly ignored. Staying under the care of a physician with whom you are uncomfortable impairs healing and health, both physical and mental.

Communicating with Your Physicians

Being told you have cancer inevitably brings a disorienting combination of disbelief, anxiety, fear, anger, and sadness. You feel as if you are in a bad dream. We protect ourselves from this onslaught of unwanted information and emotion by distancing ourselves from reality, the mental equivalent of what the hedgehog does when it feels endangered: It rolls into a ball to protect itself from what threatens it. The medical profession describes this as *dissociation*.

There are several reasons for this reaction. You may have been feeling fine when the diagnosis was presented to you. This is quite common with breast cancer, early bowel and prostate cancer, and most skin cancers. We think we are well, and the diagnosis comes out of the blue during a routine checkup or an examination for some other, probably unrelated, complaint.

Other times, with some lymphomas or early multiple myeloma, a person knows he or she is not feeling top-notch, is low in energy, a little off the normal routine, but rationalizes the change as nothing serious and even recalls prior times of feeling less than well.

Doctors as People

Strangely, your anxieties may feed on your physician's emotional discomfort in having to deliver the diagnosis to you. Doctors are into healing and curing. If they are sensitive and caring individuals, they face the consequences of your illness with shared pain. A doctor has a certain amount of anxiety and, despite training and experience, channels it by rushing you through tests with little time to question, discuss, and absorb what is going on. You may feel your doctor is becoming more abrupt, less warm, extremely businesslike. What objective medical information you are getting may be overwhelmed by the anxiety of the moment—your doctor's as well as your own!

You and Your Doctors

The feelings of the moment are fed by an unavoidable question: Is this really happening to me? And by the sense that somehow your own body has betrayed you, that something out of sight and hearing is happening inside you that threatens your existence. It is a terrible tangle of emotions, requiring a leap of faith to accept the diagnosis even as you question it.

In a way, having a lump you can feel, unusual soreness, backaches, or headaches that won't go away makes the cancer diagnosis easier to accept. But one way or another, no matter how cancer presents itself, we all engage in dissociation as a protective psychological reaction.

Dissociation, as inevitable as it is, takes you in the wrong direction. It must be overcome. You must direct the energies consumed by your anxiety toward getting back in control. Oddly, accepting the diagnosis gives you power; denying what is true also denies you control.

There are reasonable, objective facts out there, and you need to use them to integrate all the information that suddenly faces you. Your state of mind, plus the complicated, unfamiliar nature of the information you are hearing, severely limits the amount of information you retain. It also renders your memory highly selective based on fluctuations in attention because of anger, fear, and anxiety, as well as selective attention and remembering based on not hearing and not recalling things you don't want to hear. You need a prop to help you.

The prop I introduce at my seminars is a pad of paper with pencil. Have it with you every time you meet with a doctor or a member of the medical team. Write down your questions and concerns ahead of time. Then ask the questions and express your concerns. Write down what you are told. Explain that you are doing so as a way of ensuring that you get your information straight.

Studies show that rarely more than 20 percent of the information shared by your physician in the diagnostic period, during treatment reviews, or at meetings during which treatment plans are changed is retained clearly and accurately. Writing down what you are told helps minimize such dramatic losses of information. The possibility of misunderstandings is reduced. Having a friend or family member with you to write down what is shared and to review it with you later is immensely helpful.

Some doctors are threatened by this kind of behavior. It is important that you make clear that your pad of paper and pencil are intended simply to help you get things straight. Trying to tape-record meetings is usually a bad idea. (There are some exceptions to this. The visually impaired might well use a recording.) Recordings in and of themselves do not guarantee better hearing since they just repeat the same information that has been delivered to you. The act of recording makes most physicians feel untrusted and threatened; their reactions can too often result in a restrained, less openly interested caregiver. That result does not help you at all. A physician may, under those circumstances, distance himself or herself from you, becoming extremely cautious in communicating with you and possibly even overprescribing tests to cover any possible question about clinical judgment. What we all need is information openly offered and clearly understood; this leads to mutual trust.

Some patients have the will and skill to augment the information they get from the medical team by reading. That can be valuable, even for a person who has not had the time to read much before. Your local library may have appropriate books for you. Your doctor may share some books from his own library. The U.S. Government Printing Office has pamphlets that are informative, and calling the hot line of the National Cancer Institute (1-800-4-CANCER) can alert you to many resources. (See Appendix E for some other suggestions.)

Communication in Systems of Care

Whatever you do in self-education, there is nothing to replace good communication with your doctors. Control starts there. You need to know what the oncologist and staff expect of you as a patient. They expect you to cooperate with the treatment regimens prescribed and to which you have agreed. They expect you to report when you are not feeling well and to describe those feelings to the best of your ability. They expect to hear your reactions to treatments, including unusual reactions to medications. They expect you to respect their time, whether you are part of an HMO or a fee-for-service plan, and to pay your bills if it is your obligation to do so.

Then there are your expectations. You need to know how the clinic or practice operates in a number of ways. Think about what you want to know and write down your questions. Here are a few suggestions that are reasonable for patients to ask.

- With whom and how are appointments set up?
- If you must cancel an appointment, whom do you call and how early or late can you call?
- If you have questions, whom do you ask first?
- Will they call you with test results, or do you have to initiate the communication?
- How long does it take to get results?

Find out specifically from the oncologist how to arrange for conference time with him or her when *you* need it. Find out who can explain any billing for services if you have questions. (Friction with physicians too often follows misunderstandings about bills and charges.)

Remember too that you benefit from the oncologist's knowing all he or she can about you and your family situation. Who you are is more than the sum of your lab tests. Report about your preexisting health problems, including any substance abuse—alcohol or recreational drugs—even if it occurred in the past. Disclose your physical or emotional vulnerabilities, from low back pain or migraines to sleep disorders, eating disorders, or obsessiveness.

Let your doctors know (just the headlines, not necessarily the details) if you have any major economic or family problems—huge debts, unemployment, unhappy marriage, children in chronic trouble, disabled family members, absence of family and support systems. If you regularly take over-the-counter drugs including laxatives or antihistamines, that is worth reporting. Tell them a little bit about your ways of coping with stress in general as well as with fatigue, irritability, anger, and pain.

Not all of this information can be exchanged in a first meeting, but the sooner an easy communication is established, the better off you are. The more the doctor knows about you and the more you understand how the practice operates, the better off both of you will be. That is the foundation you need. If only you could stop there.

Case Manager for Yourself

Often, you may have to consult with other specialists. This brings its own problems. You may assume then that what one of your doctors knows all of them know. Not so. While they are all part of *your* team, they do not necessarily check with one another. You may, as a matter of fact, be told something by one specialist and find he or she has not communicated the information to others who should know. You may well have to be the bridge to get everyone operating with the same data. You may end up being an "air traffic controller" of information, even your own translator of information or instructions. To switch the label to a more medical one, you must often become your own case manager. Acting as your own case manager may be particularly important when your cancer requires surgery.

Surgeons

Unfortunately, and as a broad generalization, communications with surgeons are often the source of most dissatisfaction for patients. Today surgeons tend to be less hurried and more willing to explain procedures than they were ten years ago. Nonetheless, all too often surgeons function a bit like the college athletic coach—aggressive in encouraging action while minimizing the effects of the injuries received. Few of them have ever experienced anesthesia or surgery; therefore, they may well suffer from significant limits to their empathy.

Surgeons' attitudes grow naturally out of their training—more technique and technology than personal relations—and their own belief that the best possible outcome may derive from their efforts. Because surgeons wish that success rests in their hands, they often convey an energetic optimism that makes you feel good and keeps fear in check. In addition, with surgeons there tends to be more of a need to protect themselves from emotional involvement with their patients than we see with other physicians. They need to hold some distance, some separation, to be able to intrude on the body's integity through surgery—a high-stress task.

That is why it is important for you to understand that surgeons do sometimes miscommunicate about the aftereffects of surgery. They unwittingly set you up for anger directed at yourself and feelings of discouragement. They do this by minimizing the physical, physiological, and emotional aftereffects of anesthesia and of surgery. Recovery from all but the most minor surgery and local anesthesia takes much longer than the healing of surface wounds. Patience with healing takes mental preparation if you are to avoid inappropriate expectations and minimize relapses. Return to normal energy levels (physical and mental), normal mobility, and normal flexibility takes, in my experience, two to five times longer than what most surgeons state to their patients.

This is especially so if the surgery involves open entry (as opposed to laparoscopic entry) into the abdominal cavity. As a consequence of the surgeon's efforts to be a cheerleading coach, he or she minimizes the recovery time. The result is logical and inevitable. The patient starts wondering what else is wrong that healing is so slow, and depression and anxiety can follow. So, if you need surgery, protect yourself from this sequence of false hope followed by true misery.

The best protection you may have is getting the name of three or four others who have had similar surgery. Telephone them and ask about their recovery time. Your physician and/or the local American Cancer Society can help get the names of people who are willing to talk to you. Nurses can also serve as an information resource, providing more realistic information on recovery time. (Don't run back to the doctor saying the nurse says it is going to take longer to recover! That causes needless conflict. Just accept that more often than not the nurse will be on the mark.) The name of the game is being realistic. Realistic information allows you to rehearse expectations in your mind. Realistic information allows you to plan your activities more responsibly. Realistic information prevents needless anxiety, depression, and disappointment.

How to Work with Nurses and Other Medical Staff

A major ally in your effort to avoid unhelpful attitudes and conditions may well be a nurse. Nurses, in many ways, hold complex medical systems together and often are the primary communicators for patients and families. Most physicians recognize their dependence on nurses, rely on them, and trust them. This has not always been the case and is not always the case even today. But increasingly we—doctors and nurses—work together in a productive, reinforcing way that makes us better able to provide support to the patient. (Some physicians and HMOs employ physician's assistants, who generally have two years of training after high school, instead of nurses. They are licensed in some states. What I've said about nurses applies to these professionals as well.)

Nurses as Advocates and Educators

For your own good, develop a positive relationship, if you can, with the main nurse at the clinic, medical center, or practice you are working with. A nurse can become the essential interpreter and guide through the medical maze, an advocate, a source of both general and specific information to you, as well as a frequent source of supportive emotional care. Let your nurses know your level of interest in participating in your own care. Do not be afraid to ask questions of them or check with them about medicines, dosages, and your understanding of your doctor's instructions.

My only caution to you is that you not turn to the "friendliest face," accepting information and guidance on the basis of charm alone. Personal warmth, interest, and the ability to communicate are vital, but they must be viewed in the context of knowledge and training.

You will deal with nurses with different levels of training, and it is important for you to understand the variations. If you are not certain what a nurse's background is, don't be shy about asking. You may be dealing with a licensed practical nurse (L.P.N.) who has only a high school diploma plus a year of training. The L.P.N. may be helpful, caring, and informative, but only to his or her level of understanding.

The registered nurse (R.N.), the one we usually think of when we use that word, has ordinarily finished high school and had three years of training in nursing. Some nurses receive a bachelor of science in nursing degree (B.S.N.) after four or five years in college training. Some go on for a master's degree (M.S.N.) and some become clinical specialists (C.S), also called nurse practitioners. After receiving basic credentials, a clinical specialist has focused on one area of nursing—pediatrics, emergency medicine, psychiatry, or oncology, for example. Some nurses hold a Ph.D., but few of them provide direct care; you are not likely to run into one except in administrative, health policy, or research roles.

Medical Support Staff

Other staff you may deal with include receptionists, appointment secretaries, and technicians who may draw blood, help with mammograms, arteriograms, CAT scans, x-rays, and MRIs. Each of them can make your life pleasant or unpleasant in greater or lesser ways.

If they themselves are poorly supervised by your doctor, or if they have been treated disrespectfully or indifferently by doctors or other supervisors, they may well in turn treat you in a brusque and insensitive manner.

Caroline was steamed that her MRI could be scheduled only at 7:00 P.M. It meant rearranging family and work responsibilities, and that was no small matter for her. She arrived five minutes early, signed in as directed, and was ready at the appointed hour. She waited twenty minutes without explanation or apology and then was ordered around in a rude manner by the technician. By the time she got home after 9:00 P.M., she was famished, angry, and exhausted.

If you are treated that way, first see if you can, on your own, turn the behavior around, just as you might with anyone who behaves offensively. These are people, after all, just like you and me. Their moods and behavior can be changed. Start right, giving others the individual attention you would want. Recognize them as people by looking them in the eye when you say hello. Remind them of who you are—they see many people and may forget your name. If you have energy and it does not feel too awkward or forced, chat with them briefly (even superficially) asking how they are, how their day has been. If they have a picture of a child or a pet in sight, ask about it. Maybe some event (sports, entertainment, the weather) is worth commenting on, in order to put a friendly face on your relationship. It is generally worth the try. They—the aides and technicians, less well paid than many in the health care system—are people too, and your interest in them, if not intrusive, can make them more gentle and concerned caregivers.

If your efforts fail, and offensive, impersonal behavior continues, remember that you are a *purchaser of services*, not a beggar. Complain. Tell the person you don't like how you are being treated. You do not need to accept inappropriate, rough, continuously insensitive behavior. If nothing else works, tell a supervisor or your doctor. Many hospitals have a patient's advocate, an *ombudsman*, who is authorized to receive and act on complaints from patients. Hospitals also must answer to county and state health licensing agencies.

Be in Control

Be in control, stand up for yourself, and do not permit yourself to be a victim. Understand as you raise questions about how you are being treated that everyone you deal with is human and thus imperfect. Fatigue, distractions, and family problems all affect how individuals on your medical team handle their responsibilities on any given day, at any specific hour. Even in illness, you need to be sensitive to others, of course, but a pattern of unhelpful behavior can never be excused and need not be tolerated. Ask decently for better treatment, and if you do not get it, find yourself another medical team. That will rarely be necessary, but if it is, don't hesitate to take control by changing to another practice or doctor if that is possible. I am not recommending frivolous doctor shopping and bouncing from one doctor or clinic to another for the least real or imagined slight. That is self-defeating. Use common sense during an uncommon time in your life. Continuity is important, but so are comfort and confidence.

Stay in Control

A patient often assumes that the physician's office or a clinic is well organized, focused on the patient's needs, and that one is likely to be quite like another. Not true. Many offices simply grew without planning or reference to the experience of others. They may simply reflect a doctor's own style and idiosyncrasies. A few, and I hope an increasing number, are planned with the consumer and the medical staff in mind. Some are more accommodating and sensitive than others. Ironically, there are several things about the pressures of managed care that could result in making practices both more alike and more predictable. The need to document problems and treatments and to give care to as many patients as quickly as possible and the growth of business-directed practice management may help smooth out the unevenness.

Understanding the System

What is important is for you to figure out early just what you are dealing with, what kind of system you are caught up in. The challenge is to make the system work for you as well as you can. This is our old theme of taking control. For example, do not assume that others will remember to instruct you about anything. Great distress can be generated by a lack of understanding of the billing system, including out-of-network payments, the appointment system, the record and reporting systems.

Over and over I hear frustration in the voices of the people I see because reports from their doctor of a scan or other studies are missing. Over and over I hear complaints that a patient has had to wait many days for results of reports, which the patient anticipates with fear or hope, or maybe both. You yourself may have arrived at an appointment to find that your most recent scan is not there, that the latest lab test results aren't in your folder. What is so vital to you seems of so little concern to others that anger inevitably follows. And today there is always the possibility that you will sense cost containment is of greater concern to a medical practice than your health.

So what can you do? First, find out if your clinic or doctor has an established system for reporting the results of lab tests, studies, and procedures. Then ask to be instructed in its use. For example, sometimes a clinical nurse specialist carries out the task of reporting results, other times reliance is placed on voice mail, and sometimes a doctor insists that only he or she can convey that information to you. Once you've learned this about the system you are participating in, ask how long before the results will be available when a test, scan, or procedure is completed. Then call at the appropriate time, saying in an inquiring tone: "I was told the results would be in today. I wondered if they have arrived." If they aren't in, simply ask when they will be. Be persistent but not confrontational, remembering that your calm tone will likely elicit an interested, calm response.

Because nothing is more irritating than arriving for an appointment to find that a crucial bit of information is missing, call a day or so before your appointment to inquire of the appropriate person (usually a nurse or physician's assistant) whether the test or study results are in. Again, be gentle and firm rather than demanding or difficult. Your call may be just the reminder the office needs.

Making Your Records Work for You

Medical records will be part of your comfort or your distress in the health care system. While the records belong to the physician, clinic, or hospital, you have a right not only to see them but to have copies of them, including x-rays, CAT scans, and MRIs. Having the right to them, however, is not the same thing as demanding copies of everything. That just becomes a source of dust collection in your home and a bewildering impractical accumulation of paper. Records are essential to your continuity of care and a quality assurance tool for all involved in your care.

So, you should keep a file at home in which you have a copy of the original diagnostic reports, all treatment plans, all hospital discharge summaries, and the reports from all major studies made on your case. Those records give you both information and the freedom to consult with others as you see fit or as you are advised to do so. An alternative to this recommendation for some involves having the trusted family physician be the recipient of such summaries and reports.

If you have more than one physician prescribing medications for you, keep a complete list of the medications and their dosages in that file and note any side effects you experience, including their frequency and precisely what they are. You should also list all over-the-counter (OTC) medications as well as herbal, homeopathic, or naturopathic substances you take.

You should share that list with your primary-care physician. Much discomfort, even outright illness, is caused every year because of complex interactions of multiple drugs and substances. Occasionally it is not the interaction but a new substance itself, even a common one, that causes problems. Some vitamins in excessive amounts can be poisonous. Some mineral supplements are impure and can produce toxic conditions, such as mercury poisoning from some dolomite sources. Antibiotics, as vital as they are, can make some people very sick, even producing changes in psychological functioning. Only you have the overriding interest in keeping accurate track of side effects; advocacy for yourself should be your highest priority. That does not come naturally or easily for many of us. Standing up for yourself becomes even more of a challenge when you are feeling low in energy and mood.

Making Sure Your Needs Are Met

In fact, most people worry, even in illness, about making a nuisance of themselves, but you need to know how to get special attention when you require it. This may involve an extra appointment for reassurance about something, a consultation about pain management, a discussion of quality-of-life concerns. As early as possible in your relationship with your specialist, clarify how to get that attention when you need it. Your oncologist, after all, should be the best equipped to teach you what symptoms to worry about and which ones can be safely ignored.

Demands on your physician's time have escalated dramatically during the last ten years. Reports to insurance companies and to the government take time. The computer is wonderful for storing data, but that takes time, too; data retrieval is time consuming as well. A chronic condition for all physicians these days is the feeling of spending more time with paperwork and computers than with patients, and the doctors don't like it any better than you do.

Learn how your system works concerning lab reports and special study reports (x-rays, bone scans, sonograms, CAT scans, MRIs, etc.). Where are these reports done, and how long before they are available to the office and to you? How quickly can you get a copy of the report? Who provides an explanation and is available for discussion of the report, and how promptly after the results are in do those discussions happen? You may be willing to have all that information given to you over the phone, although I strongly believe that significant information, either positive or negative, is worth an appointment, a trip to the doctor's office, and should be communicated in person.

Mastering Information

Information is a blessing and vital. But misinformation can be devastating, because it festers and distorts and frightens. Bits and pieces do not inform. A conversation is often overheard and partially understood by patients. When this involves statements about prognosis and longevity, the potential for misunderstanding becomes very high, and elevated anxiety in all of us interferes with clear thinking and memory.

Check what you have heard. That is why it is so crucial that you know to whom you should turn so that you can quickly resolve any doubts about what you have heard. You should not have to hear anything about your illness by accident or because two staff people are talking in a manner that can be overheard. If complaints are in order, know ahead of time where you should direct them. There is no absolute system that works in all instances. The answers to these questions are specific to your doctor's office or the clinic providing your health care. Master that system through asking and learning, and you become less a victim of both your disease and the medical system.

Help with Self-Care

The big events in the course of an illness are obviously important, but don't ignore the details of some seemingly lesser concerns of self-care. Who, in the system you are using, will provide this kind of information? Self-care includes dental health, exercise, nutrition, prevention of infections including hepatitis and tuberculosis, and handling of colds and more serious infections. Knowing what changes in your body rhythms, such as sleep or energy levels, need attention and which ones can be ignored is important. Knowing what changes in symptoms, including your capacity to focus and think clearly, should be of concern and which are not significant—all of this becomes part of the learning process in mastering your role as a cancer patient. You need to know what symptoms are appropriate to report to your physician and which ones you can ignore.

Help with Self-Image

You also need to face issues of changes in the way you look that are created by chemotherapy, radiation therapy, or surgery. These include temporary as well as long-term changes. Many of the changes are experienced as disfigurements by the individuals in whom they have occurred. Sometimes they are seen as disfigurements by others. Hair loss, changes in hair color and texture, changes in skin color and texture because of radiation, changes in skin sensitivity as the result of radiation, scars from surgery, new ways of eliminating body wastes, surgical losses of parts of the body, significantly decreased energy, changes in sharpness and clarity of thinking, increased self-consciousness about normal body functions—all present emotional challenges to a cancer patient.

An extraordinary amount of information exists to help you deal with such changes. Some of this information is provided in the resources of Appendix E of this book. More direct forms of information should be available through your doctor's office or clinic.

Let Your Voice Be Heard

The reality of modern hospitals, not the sanitized image we all see on television, and of medical technology is scary. Monitors, electrically driven intravenous devices for fluids, medicines, and feedings, catheters implanted in the chest wall, MRI machines, operating rooms with lights and sinks and equipment contribute to a sense of a hard-metal universe, dehumanized, but with you at its center, seemingly without control over anything. Add to all that the sounds and smells of that unfamiliar environment, and you become an uneasy visitor to a place where things are done to you, though admittedly on your behalf. Questioned, poked, prodded, stuck, dressed, undressed, peered into over and over, by doctors and nurses you know and often by strangers you don't, you lose your privacy and your sense of control.

To survive these intrusions, do your best to inquire, to learn about and to familiarize yourself with all your experiences. Knowledge allows trust. Knowledge also allows you to speak up if you suspect errors, and errors are occasionally made.

All the different chemotherapeutic agents have different effects. Your doctors and nurses can tell you about some of them.

You can also read about them in readily available free brochures from the National Cancer Institute.

Radiation therapy starts with simulations and often dye tattoos, which are placed on the body to guide the radiation therapist. Stress is increased by waiting your turn for the radiation and the fatigue that eventually occurs as you progress in a radiation therapy series. Specific areas of hair loss and local skin swelling and redness may also contribute to your stress.

How do you deal with the repeated needle punctures by individuals who are less expert than they should be in drawing blood? How do you deal with rough handling or handling that shows little concern or compassion for you as an individual? How do you deal with the fear of intrusive and strange-sounding procedures such as bronchoscopies, gastrostomies, colonoscopies? How do you mobilize the support of families? How do you influence the system when it is being unhelpful to you?

You simply must face these experiences directly and not let fatigue, fear, or embarrassment keep you silent. You need to question and ask for explanations until you understand. When some procedure makes no sense or you see no benefit in it, *you do not have to agree to it.* Feel free to seek second opinions even about whether certain tests or procedures are necessary. And remember, your self-respect, at the very least, requires that you stand up for yourself, complaining, verbally and in writing, if you are handled in an uncaring, rough, or hurtful fashion. You will, through all of this, empower yourself. And through empowerment you enhance your capacity to heal.

3 Increasing Your Healing Skills

PEOPLE WHO ATTEND my "Living with Cancer" seminars often ask me to speak about stress management but rarely ask me to discuss the broader subject of health maintenance. I do anyway. Perhaps it seems silly to talk about other health matters when you are fighting cancer. It really is not. In fact it is even more important than ever that you do those things that permit and encourage your body to function well.

You simply cannot fight your cancer effectively if healthy living choices, quite within your control, are ignored. Proper concern allows your body to use its energies and other resources for optimal healing. You need that, and you can have it, if you will follow several simple rules.

Let's list some elements of an ideal health maintenance routine, discussing many of them in the sections that follow. The elements include:

- regular exercise
- regular life rhythms (sleep, wake/activity, elimination)—medical science now documents that Ben Franklin had the right idea when he wrote in *Poor Richard's Almanac,* "Early to bed, and early to rise, makes a man healthy, wealthy, and wise."
- good stress management
- good personal hygiene, including oral/dental health
- conservative use of alcohol and caffeine; avoidance of tobacco and its associated toxins
- appropriate nutrition
- opportunity and freedom to express your sexuality in ways appropriate to your age and circumstances
- active engagement of your mind in things that you care about
- caring involvement with others and with the community in a way that makes you feel needed
- assessment of your vulnerabilities
- having a sense of predictability and control
- examination of your attitude and psychological state
- occupying a basically pleasing environment
- having access to reasonable economic and material resources
- having joyful moments
- opening your mind to a sense of connectedness with living things and life beyond yourself (a form of spirituality)

Movement and Health

Decades ago exercise stopped being a natural part of many Americans' lives. Most of us no longer walk as often as we ride, we don't plow the fields to grow what we eat; most of us don't perform any regular manual labor. Our society talks a lot about exercise and does so for good reason. To remain as healthy as they can, our bodies need exercise.

Our Two Circulatory Systems

Blood pumped by the heart as it circulates through the body delivers oxygen and nutrients, takes away waste products, and helps with clotting and wound healing. But there is another circulatory system that complements our blood. The lymphatic system is actually the main vehicle for the immune system's functioning. Unlike the relation of the heart to blood circulation, there is no special pump that helps the lymphatic system circulate its fluid, the lymph. It relies primarily on muscle activity to provide energy for its flow. Without exercise lymph flow decreases through our tissues. This means that we have to exercise to get the most out of our immune systems. (I really cannot emphasize exercise, which means movement of our bodies, enough. This certainly doesn't mean, however, that you have to undertake strenuous new activities or achieve extraordinary competence in some sport.)

To clearly understand our need for exercise, think of a city. Roads and railroads bring in supplies and take out wastes. Underground pipes carry water, liquid wastes, electricity, gas, and steam. Without all of these roads and underground conduits, the city could not live. If they get slowed down, the city will slow down (as in a power brownout); if they get blocked, the city will start to die. Exercise is the process that keeps our human roads and conduits (blood and lymphatic systems) unblocked, freely flowing. Without exercise, we "sludge," slow down, become unhealthy, begin to die.

The seven people in the Wednesday night support group all had different cancers. One evening, Doris and Sam spoke with great distress about the fatigue they were experiencing. Melissa, another group member, spoke of how she had discovered, after several weeks of making

herself exercise regularly, that her fatigue had diminished and she was coping better with it. The problem, the challenge, she found was doing something she was not used to.

Exercise

Health maintenance exercise does not mean high-impact aerobics, jogging, or cheetahlike exercise in intense bursts. Serious walking may be enough, just as it was for our hunter-gatherer ancestors one or two hundred thousand years ago. Our bodies have evolved little since then, though our lifestyles certainly have changed. Walking, frequently long distances, is still our most natural form of exercise, and we should combine it with stretching as a minimum health maintenance routine.

Movement enhances health. No matter what your level of illness, you must engage in some form of exercise. No matter how bad you feel, move and stretch regularly and to the extent you can. Listen to your body, however, for it will protest if you are overdoing it. Even if you are limited to a wheelchair or bed, you can engage in some form of exercise, using stretching and the movement of muscles that can be moved. Work gently, gradually toward making your exercise a regular part of your self-care program as well as increasing the amount you do. It is clear that exercise to a level that is appropriate for our body improves our capacity to heal as well as enhances our emotional sense of well-being.

Frequently professional physical therapy assistance with a plan of movement and exercise makes a significant contribution to recovery. Physical therapy is important to any patient who has had surgical interventions, and particularly to breast cancer patients, amputees, and those with chronic pain. Physical therapy helps you, if you have special needs, understand how to use and position your body considering the changes that have occurred after surgery or radiation treatments or in the context of chronic pain. A physical therapist will help you correct any unhelpful postures and movements. Therapists teach appropriate range of motion and strengthening exercises of the neck, extremities, and torso. A consultation with a registered physical therapist can help improve circulation and, as a result, healing through individually tailored exercises. It is often useful to take a friend or relative to physical therapy sessions so that once you are back home he or she can help you practice some of the techniques demonstrated and prescribed by the physical therapist.

Your circulation can also be improved through various massage techniques. Most forms of massage have direct effects on the movement, contraction, and relaxation of skeletal muscles. Current research indicates that massage has positive effects on the body's healing responses as well as on mood states.

Understanding Stress

Brenda, one of my patients, said to me one day, "The way some of my friends react when they learn I have cancer makes me think that all the stress in my life gave me cancer. Is that so?"

Brenda asked a question that I am asked more often than any other, and that suggests that there are profound misunderstandings about stress among many cancer patients. It is important to eliminate those misunderstandings.

Stress is a normal part of life. It is with you every day from childhood on up—in cuts, bruises, colds, tests, and reports in school. As we grow, there are inevitable conflicts with parents and siblings, with classmates and teachers. All of that leads to stress.

As adolescents, we have the unavoidable stress of evolving sexual identity, dating, courtship, and the responsibilities of setting out on our own. As adults we all face stress in dealing with supervisors and colleagues at work, with clerks in stores, in traffic jams, even with spouses, children, and friends. So what does the word *stress* really mean? *Stress* refers to events and forces that have some impact on us in a way that demands adjustment by us—physically, psychologically, or both. The adjustment may or may not involve action visible to others. There is virtually no stress-free existence in the best of times, and responding to stress is just part of living. Some of us handle it better than others.

Stress and Illness

New stresses of an intense sort become constant and unwelcome companions with the diagnosis of cancer. These stresses are inevitable, inescapable, and may be unrelenting. They come at you from virtually all directions and may produce anxiety, tension, sleep problems, and fear. Your life, which once had some predictable familiarity, is suddenly filled with questions.

The questions start with the illness. Is it real? Is the diagnosis right? The doctor you have trusted you now may doubt, at least a little bit. Have the doctor and the team of consultants and staff selected the best treatments? Will treatment permit a reasonably normal life, or will the life rhythms you are accustomed to be interrupted? Will changes be painful or devastating or reasonably tolerable? Will the treatments work? For most of us, the diagnosis drives us into an entirely new area of knowledge (or ignorance). It is disconcerting.

Then there is the social aspect of the diagnosis. Who do you tell? What do you tell? When do you tell? How will family and friends react? How, indeed, do you want them to react—with gloom and tears, with real optimism, or with false cheer? They will be just as unsure as you, maybe more so, about how they should behave. As the patient, you ironically may have to be educator and guide to others. These roles impose additional stress on you.

Joanne may or may not be speaking for her husband, Ted, who is the one with cancer. She said heatedly, "This is hell, this waiting to know the extent of Ted's cancer. I just want the treatments started now so we

can get on with our lives." Even waiting for a complete diagnosis and a treatment plan can become a stress.

Even routine things are hard to handle. Awaiting the readings of every lab test, the results of every checkup is stress before and stress after. What will the tests show? Why hasn't the doctor called? Why aren't the test results back? Why do you have to wait an hour or a day or a week without a definitive answer? Why? Why? Why? What do the results, now that you've got them, really mean? This litany of uncertainties seems pretty horrible, doesn't it?

Beyond that, few of us escape the economic worries that come with illness. For those who are working and dependent on that income, the specter of inability to continue steady labor looms. How you will make ends meet is a question that won't go away. Beyond that, there are inevitable questions of how expensive treatment will be and whether your health insurance will cover all the costs. You face an economic landscape filled with boulders and potholes; it is distressing.

Finally, of course, there is the stress that arises from pain. Surgery and radiation are never fun, never pleasant, and almost always associated with some pain, as are some cancers. Sometimes the pain is acute and of short duration. For some patients pain may be minimally intense but chronic; for others pain is severe and chronic. Pain brings questions. If pain is less today, will it be worse tomorrow? Is there any way that you can control your pain? It all adds up to stress and then more stress.

Handling Stress

But wait a minute. You don't have to surrender to stress. You can fight to regain control. You can work at handling stress as you have done before in your life with both minor and serious problems. You do not have to accept the victim role. *Victim*, by the way, comes from the Latin word, *victima,* which meant "beast for sacrifice." *You are not that.* You are a human being with the resources and ability to bear up under pain, distress, loss, and injury. You can manage stress because you were created as one of the planet's most adaptable beings. That management begins with understanding how humans are made, what stress means in our lives, and what stresses do to our bodies.

Let me start with my conclusions and then give you some human history and physiology in support of them.

We handle stress successfully when we learn to modulate our responses, avoiding overreaction to whatever situation we are in. Survival and well-being require that we deal with reality as it is, neither losing hope nor seizing on false dreams. We need to channel our energies and our state of mind in the direction of coping, seeking new accommodation and control rather than accepting our new realities. There is no magic about learning to be calm in the face of major challenges. Being positive in outlook may not be easy, but it is not impossible.

It does not take a genius to figure out how to improve how we handle stress. Each one of us has that potential and can learn how to enhance our skills. You *can* control your responses to the many stresses of your life.

Our Bodies, Our Cells

First, consider how the human body is constructed. At the most basic level, the body is made up of small, vibrant structures called *cells*, which begin with the first divisions of a fertilized egg. Those cells become specialized into tissues—bone, muscles, nerves, skin, blood and immune systems, plus organs such as the liver, heart, kidneys, and pancreas. Thus the human body is a group of collaborating, specialized cells that communicate with each other to make the individual. That whole feeds, excretes, reproduces, and also interacts with the environment.

Our cells communicate within our bodies through both chemical and electrical means—hormones, neurotransmitters, and other small molecules called *polypeptides* on the one hand and nerves and other conducting tissues on the other. Few laypeople understand human biology in detail, and you certainly should not worry if you don't. A general understanding of the body's complexity is probably enough. That understanding reminds us that miracles do occur all the time in each of us—billions of cells communicating in an individual whole you see whenever you look into a mirror.

We are a wondrously complex chemical and electrical system whose constant cascade of invisible interactions constitutes our functioning and determines our physical well-being. You can affect that process with your mind as well. I am not talking about miracles of cure—though that may happen—but I am suggesting that how you handle stress can make a significant difference in your life.

Physical Reactions to Stress

Let us consider an everyday event. You start across a street, and a car suddenly turns in your direction. You pick it up in your peripheral vision and jump back toward the sidewalk. The car doesn't hit you, and you don't stumble. In essence nothing has happened, but your blood pressure has changed, your heart rate has changed, the circulation of your blood to your extremities has increased, and many more subtle chemical and electrical alterations in terms of hormones and neurotransmitters have occurred. You may curse the driver, shake your fist, or do nothing.

We respond in many ways all the time to perceived events as well as to the things that actually touch us. The example I just cited is one kind of negative perceived event. Others may be an upcoming deadline, a disagreement with a spouse, a criticism from a boss. Positive perceived events can be anticipating seeing someone we love, taking a vacation, receiving a compliment. Things that directly touch us can be the positive experiences of a vacation, a wonderful meal, a massage, an exciting concert. Negative experiences might be a disappointing evening, a car accident, an injury, nonelective surgery.

Another perspective on human activity, referred to earlier, is relevant to understanding stress. The human body is today quite like what it was more than 150,000 years ago. We have not significantly evolved physically beyond the hunter-gatherers we once were. We react today when challenged much as they did. In biology, medicine, and psychology, we refer to this form of response as the fight-or-flight reaction.

The tiger that leaped out at our long-gone forebears is itself long gone. Today being told that we have cancer is our tiger, the modern threat to our existence. A lab test that does not show the favorable response you hoped for makes you respond in a modified way physically as if you were being attacked by a tiger. A relative or friend who says something insensitive or even unkind is a leaping or stalking tiger. Our bodies respond to all these situations as though we were being attacked. We are constructed to react to all experiences with cascades of chemical and electrical events that mobilize us to survive through increased activity; this often meant to run or to fight.

A third aspect of stress involves duration. An illustration comes also from the animal kingdom. The cheetah is a magnificent large wild cat, probably our fastest four-legged creature. It can run up to sixty-five miles an hour while chasing its prey. That is extraordinarily stressful for its body, but within tolerable limits. However, it can run that fast only in short spurts, maybe three or four minutes at a time. If forced to run faster or longer, it will falter, get sick, possibly even die. Like the cheetah, we must modulate the length of time we are in a fight-or-flight mode; we need to get beyond immediate challenges and acute threats. We need to shift to a state of mind and a physiological state that allows our personal chemical-electrical system to rebalance itself, to direct our energies toward healing and repair.

For many individuals the cumulative effects of years of poor self-regulation of stress responses, of continuing the fight-or-flight pattern without a break works against the healing and repair activities that require quieter moments. This may be a significant influencing factor in the development of chronic disease states. For cancer patients, it clearly influences responses to treatments of the illness.

Some Techniques of Stress Management

"Wanda and I handle stress so differently. It's ironic that we both have chronic illnesses now; she with her MS and I with my cancer. Maybe the fact that I was in a prisoner-of-war camp in Asia when I was eight years old makes the difference. I became good at putting out of my mind my hunger, my loneliness, the scary things I saw. She just can't let anything go. She keeps thinking over and over about everything. For me, if something unhappy or scary happens, I deal with it as best I can, but then it's gone from my mind. It takes an effort to even remember how I felt about it."

Much hope can be derived from employing good stress management skills. This section illustrates the essential ones for you. If you use them well, your sense of control and well-being will improve.

Self-Inventory

As the shock of a cancer diagnosis begins to decrease, it is critical, I believe, that you do a self-inventory. You need to evaluate how well you are responding to the increased stress. Move from high gear, if that is where you are, sit back, and try to look dispassionately at your actions. A good beginning is to ask yourself how you are dealing with the problems of your day-to-day life. Also, what state of mind are you in? Is the choke on your personal motor pulled out to full-throttle position (fight or flight) so that you cannot even turn off your worrying thoughts? After answering these questions, do a general inventory of your stress management skills:

- How good are you at being aware of your physical state, particularly fatigue and tension?
- Can you, on your own, truly relax?
- Does your thinking style improve your sense of control?
- Do you know how to modify your environment to one that is optimum for healing?
- Do you actively use techniques that mobilize healing responses?

Self-Regulatory Skills and Biofeedback

Having done your self-inventory, consider biofeedback administered by a trained, certified therapist as a way of objectively measuring your physical levels of stress as well as your natural capacity to relax yourself. *Biofeedback* means just what the word implies: feedback to the observing individual of selected measurable expressions of biologic functioning. By using electronic sensors that measure muscle tension, skin temperature, sweat gland activity, blood pressure, heart rate, the rate of breathing, and brain wave activity, therapists can learn whether you can read your body responses well and whether you have the capacity to alter these responses with your thoughts in a way that is appropriate for the situation: for example, increased alertness or increased relaxation.

Through biofeedback training you can be taught to increase your skills in modulating your physical responses to stress. Even those individuals who have had transcendental meditation or yoga training find biofeedback useful. Everyone benefits from at least a one-time evaluation, because no other reliable way exists to quickly, objectively evaluate self-regulatory skills.

To alter physiologic responses with our thoughts is a skill that we all potentially have. It can be learned by everyone through training and regular practice. Past bad habits of overreactions to stressful situations are a luxury you can ill afford when faced with cancer. Fortunately, stress management training is much like learning to ride a bicycle or learning to scuba dive, in that once those skills are basically mastered they are with you forever.

So, biofeedback is just what it describes itself as: electronic machines sensing responses from muscles, sweat glands, and blood to measure physical responses to different situations, including physical and mental stress, as well as relaxation. Most of the time we measure the muscles over the face and neck, temperature and sweat gland activity in the hands. The electrodes used are in contact only with the surface of the skin.

We know that the muscles of the face and neck are highly responsive to emotional states and stresses. We also know that peripheral temperature as well as sweat gland activity respond in particular directions when an individual is feeling stressed. Normal responses for people of different ages and sexes are well known. Thus, based on an evaluation, you can learn whether you are within the normal range of reactions and whether you have reasonable skills in recognizing your physical states and in altering those states at will. If not, a certified biofeedback therapist can work with you to improve your capacity to calm yourself down, or, if you are a person with a "hair trigger" system (also called a *hot reactor*), you can receive training to dampen intense, dramatic reactions to negative or frightening experiences.

Children are quicker to learn self-regulation skills than adults. Using biofeedback, they can often master skills within two to four weeks of training. Adults often take four to five months. Much of the practice needed to attain good self-regulation skills can be done using training audiotapes specifically tailored for each individual. Office training sessions run by professionals and home practice guided by the audiotapes instruct you in techniques for using your mind (through commands to the body) to reduce muscle tension, raise skin temperature, improve breathing, and decrease sweating. Results are clearly related to how regularly you practice. Practicing once a week, for example, is a waste of time. Practice of fifteen to twenty minutes a day, seven days a week, usually produces dramatic improvement in your skills.

So, learning these techniques not only helps you engage in preventive health care but also empowers you. These techniques give you the capacity to use your mind, your will to make positive changes in physical functioning. Athletes use them, and you can, too. With feedback given to them on their swing, body posture, and tension, tennis players, golfers, and baseball players can improve their game. Learning such techniques does not have to be done in isolation. It can be done with a friend or a family member who can be with you as a coach, pacer, and encourager.

Breath Control

Few of us think about breathing as something that can be done well or poorly. We just breathe. In our culture we, in fact, often breathe improperly by raising our shoulders, not extending our abdomen, and consequently only partially expanding our chest. When that happens, our lungs are not completely filled, resulting in insufficient exchange of oxygen and inadequate waste elimination of carbon dioxide and water. Shallow breathing often comes with excitement or tension and when our bodies are in a vigilant or modified fight-or-flight state.

Slow, deep breathing, on the other hand, is something we associate correctly with relaxing, feeling calm, being in control. We fill our lungs completely. We feel less stressed. Breathing techniques are important to stress management. Our rate and depth of breathing inform the brain, through chemical and electrical signals, about how aroused and ready to do battle or flee we should be. Thus, if you are going to have major surgery, deep breathing skills can make a significant difference in how you handle your inevitable distress. We've known this for some time. In the past, though less frequently recently, hospitals routinely offered brief visits by respiration therapists to instruct patients on proper breathing techniques.

Proper breath control may seem an inconsequential bit of self-care, but it really is not. It is worth thinking about not just in anticipation of major surgery. Any procedure that involves pain or even just long periods of isolation such as radiation or an MRI or CAT scan is easier with proper breathing as a path to inducing the quieting or relaxation response.

There is considerable data that people recover from anesthesia much more quickly and have less postoperative pain and fewer complications when they not only know what to expect but also have learned proper breathing and relaxation techniques. Indeed, some studies report that, given the same medical condition and the same surgical procedure, people will leave hospitals as much as 30 percent sooner than others who have not had such training.

Special Uses of the Mind

Everything in our awareness can be said to be "of the mind." But among stress management techniques, we find certain ways of using the mind that go way beyond more accurately reading your body signals or improving your ability to down- or up-regulate your fight-or-flight responses. These uses of the mind create a setting for healing by promoting enhanced positive functioning of your chemical-electrical system. They include at least five realms: attitude, self-valuing, using joy and laughter, understanding anxiety and depression, and using ritual guided imagery.

Attitude and Self-Valuing

You should give yourself permission to discuss your illness, read the diagnostic test results, and discuss the treatments with your physician until you understand all the facts. When something doesn't make sense to you, ask for more information. The burden for helping you understand is the physician's. Keep in mind that you are smart enough to understand anything about your body if the person explaining takes the time, cares enough, and, most important, is willing to help you understand. Don't be dominated by the arrogance of others. If your doctor or others on your medical team cannot help you understand in a way that works for you, see it as their flaw, not your own. Not understanding is not good!

Denying the existence and/or the importance of pressures placed on you to function or perform constitutes an attitude guaranteed to diminish successful coping. Don't ignore the drop-off in efficiency and the drain on energy produced by uninterrupted efforts. Take note of the fatigue generated by uninterrupted work or effort of any type, physical or mental. The mental and even physical fatigue of making, arranging, and keeping doctors' appointments, keeping family and friends posted on your well-being, tracking lab tests and x-rays is considerable. Pressure in many forms can come from family, the workplace, or the community. By accepting the reality of those pressures, you're well on your way to managing them and thus improving the quality of your life.

Poor stress management is definitely occurring when you feel overwhelmed by all that is going on and see yourself unable to set goals or failing them one at a time. All of us need to have control and trust that what we expect to happen will happen—the plane we take will get us to where we're going safely; the medicine we take does what we're told it will do; the food we buy is safe, not spoiled. Thus any attitude that seeks control and expects reasonable responses from the world we live in sets a tone that promotes healing.

Joy and Laughter

You need to maintain, no matter how difficult, a sense of joy and enthusiasm for some of your activities. You cannot let life become only a series of dull events interspersed with health problems. That is a prescription for misery.

Joy is a very individual thing. It may come from talking to your African violets or a flowering cyclamen. It may be in fishing or watching birds at your feeder, drawing or painting, listening to music you love, singing to yourself, or working in your garden. It often is found in being with someone you love, child or adult. You must seek it. However you find it, make it part of your life every week.

Joy may also come from memories. Some adults associate joy only with their childhood or adolescent years, recalling long-ago experiences where time seemed to fly and the world felt very good. But joy and happiness are not the prize of youth alone. Joyful activities can be anything that helps you let go, driven no longer by the *shoulds* and *should-nots* of the world but by good feelings about good times in your life. Joy brings a relaxed state, once again different and preferable to the fight-or-flight response, and it affects your immune system in positive ways.

Laughter is hard to come by when you are ill, particularly when the diagnosis is cancer. But there has never been a more important time to laugh a little, to find the capacity to make fun of even unfunny situations, to indulge yourself in a human and a satiric view of what's happening.

Satire lets you step back, even for a few seconds, from overwhelming experiences. There are studies that indicate that humor and satire serve not only as "narrow escapes from despair" but bring about positive changes in the human system, encouraging the body to seek balance and to heal.

The diagnosis of cancer brings everyone, naturally cheerful or not, higher levels of physical and emotional exhaustion. You need to expect, accept, and respect that reality. Humor, joy, and laughter are mind skills like learning relaxation. Together they make up several of the stress management skills we need to use.

Understanding and Avoiding Depression

You need to respect the reality that part of life is having anxiety, episodes of depression, difficulty in sleeping, and moments of fear, even panic. All of that is inevitable and normal, but when prolonged, it does impair healing and needs to be dealt with. Such episodes should come and go relatively quickly. If they last as long as a week or ten days, call them to the attention of your oncologist and family physician.

How often cancer patients avoid seeking help for depression or anxiety by saying "It's bad enough that I have cancer," as though there were some stigma to being depressed or anxious! (Remember that depression may exist either with or without a conscious feeling of sadness. It is associated with a loss of motivation, a loss of interest, increased feelings of guilt, a loss of orientation toward the future, and a loss of pleasure in things or people.)

In our minds we carry images of our younger, healthier selves. Then, labeled as cancer patients, launched into treatments, we become flooded with new activities (visits to doctors, medical procedures) as well as changes, physical and emotional, social and economic, in our families and elsewhere. Overwhelmed at first, we struggle to regain a sense of control and predictability. Fatigue, irritability, and other possible side effects of the treatments (embarrassment at having a change in body image, changes in the capacities of the senses to function and sometimes in the ability to communicate, decreased sharpness of thinking, pain, disrupted sleep) makes our current reality more difficult.

With the loss of energy and health comes grieving for that loss. You grieve for the loss of the illusion of certainty and for a diminished freedom to plan. Your self-worth is diminished as you discover that the "old friends" of reason (knowing how to solve problems, plan solutions) and willpower are no longer sufficient. Anxiety and depression set in. You notice them through changes in your feelings, reactions to events, and behavior. With that anxiety and depression, your brain metabolism and chemistry have changed.

Treatment, particularly antibiotics and chemotherapy, may make brain chemistry changes worse, as do infections and unanticipated side effects, such as decreased strength and coordination. If, before the diagnosis of cancer, you suffered from a preexisting medical condition, mental health problem, or developmental problem (e.g., residual attention deficit disorder, learning disability, cerebral palsy, etc.) their influence on your day-to-day functioning may be magnified, often worsening effects on sleep pattern, anxiety, and depression. (For a few individuals this escalates to their developing a form of posttraumatic stress disorder with recurrent nightmares and flashbacks.) The reactive anxieties and depression of spouses and important others also add to your own distress.

No gold stars are given to you for suffering in silence with any of this. Know that all forms of anxiety, depression, panic attacks, and sleep disorders can be treated. Sometimes the major treatment intervention is as simple as adjusting medications that have induced the problem directly or though drug-drug interactions.

Imagery

Another skill, quite popular in recent years, is the use of imagination, or "guided imagery." Guided imagery is the use of your imagination while in a relaxed state to focus on body functions relating to healing. Using guided imagery during chemotherapy, radiation, or other therapies, for example, you visualize cancer cells being destroyed, broken into pieces and excreted, the body becoming healthier and more whole. This process of relaxing paired with creating visual images in your mind of your body getting healthier and stronger allows you to step out of the victim role and actively participate in fighting the cancer as well as in the healing process. A brief series (three to five meetings) of training sessions, either in a group or individually, with professionals is sufficient for most people.

It is important to note that research from around the world in the field of psychoneuroimmunology shows the use of imagination during a relaxed state does result in positive physical changes such as more efficient use of oxygen, decreased blood pressure, and enhanced immune system function. You can "image" yourself healing, and you can "image" your body fighting cancer. The images you come up with should not be imposed on you by others, or even given to you by others. They should be developed by you, perhaps with the help of others, using your experiences, your sense of color, sound, shape, and form. It is a very positive form of both stress management and health maintenance.

Medication and Psychotherapy

Psychopharmacologic medications—the medicines that alter anxiety, mood states, quality and quantity of thinking, energy levels, and behavior—as well as different forms of individual, couples, and family psychotherapy, and always group therapy, are other paths to improvement in stress management. When medications are administered by well-trained professionals, they may reduce symptoms and improve well-being and self-care. This route may be appropriate if anxiety, fearfulness, panic, depression, and sleep problems are patterns for you rather than just moments of dysfunction.

Patterns of dysfunction have become so much a part of life for some individuals that they have no idea what it is like to be without them. Often such individuals have accommodated to simply feeling different without realizing that they have a psychological problem. If this is true for you, you might find yourself explaining these feelings of difference, both to yourself and to others, by saying that you are simply bored or not enthusiastic or have lost your sense of humor.

You also may feel isolated, empty, lonely, and constantly irritable. You may have associated physical complaints, which can include generalized body pain or constant, specific pains of the head, chest, and back. Other physical complaints can focus on the bowels or urinary tract. If you are experiencing a pattern of dysfunction, you might discover that you feel better when you are drinking alcohol or taking self-prescribed substances, including over-the-counter medications. All of this is consistent with significant problems in psychological state.

Understand that these problems often arise over time and are both colored as well as reinforced by how you think to yourself about the experiences you are having. Such shaping of thoughts often occurs beyond conscious recognition. The result can be unhelpful styles of thinking. These styles can be anything from constant negative interpretations of experience to frequent conviction that you know what other people must be thinking without ever testing whether your assumptions are correct and a polarized "black or white" perception of events or experiences. They probably are associated with subtle changes in brain physiology, including altered patterns of neuronal communication.

There are ways of correcting such problems in thinking style through special therapy, which can be approached through self-help thought retraining workbooks or direct professional assistance from mental health professionals trained in cognitive therapy who see people individually or in groups.

When medications are needed for sleep, anxiety, or depression, learn about the side effects of the medications. Work with your prescribing physician to choose the best medication for you. Choice is made based on the speed of action, previous experiences with similar medications, and predictable side effects. Always use medications with reference to particular target symptoms—feelings, mood states, and behavior that you experience as dysfunctional and would like to see improve. Measure improvement against these target symptoms.

How Psychotherapies Can Help

How can available psychotherapies help you? When conducted by competent, licensed, well-trained professionals, psychotherapies can serve many positive purposes. They provide focused opportunities to express and examine in a nonjudgmental setting your positive and negative emotions. This can lead to reevaluation of your psychological defenses, allowing them to be modified and strengthened as needed. They provide a setting in which the responses to antianxiety and antidepressant medications can be monitored. They provide a setting in which you can learn imagery, meditation, and self-hypnotic skills.

Group therapy with other cancer patients is now recommended more and more often as part of the cancer treatment regimen, at least for the first year following diagnosis. Professionally led groups create a setting in which many things transpire: education and problem solving, including skill sharing on dealing with doctors, pain control, and other personal problems; building of bonds and support with others who are dealing with a similar illness, thus decreasing feelings of isolation and loneliness; special social skill training that cancer patients sometimes need as they encounter the reactions and behaviors of others; discussion and "detoxification" of death and dying; expression of emotions without worry about burdening friends or family members. Through it all, these gatherings create a forum in which the guiding professional can help you successfully engage in a positive restructuring of the way you think about your experiences.

Nutrition, Food, and Taste

We are overwhelmed these days with information on nutrition. It is difficult to determine what is fact, fantasy, or fad. What is clear is that food and eating are not only nourishment but also comfort and a potential reminder of protection and emotional sustenance (our being fed as infants). That has been true in every culture throughout human evolution.

We and our memories are stimulated by the color, smell, taste, texture, flavorings, and presentation of food. Food has different meanings for different people when served cold or hot, when served in community, family, or celebratory settings. Throughout the world and throughout recorded history, people have cooked for and fed others who are ill. This is experienced as caring and often an expression of love. So, the meanings and rituals of food and eating must not be ignored. Not infrequently, because of radiation and chemotherapy, the quality, even the very existence of the important rituals involving eating are seriously disrupted. If this occurs, strive to reestablish them in some form.

Food Fad Cautions

Volumes continue to be written about nutrition and diet. The greatest danger of many of them to you is the constant generation of new food fads. Such fads receive momentum from the desire of individuals to identify fountain-of-youth substances that will magically prolong healthful life. These wishes constitute major themes in Western culture over thousands of years. Some food fads turn out to have substance. An example is the fad started in the nineteenth century by clergyman Sylvester Graham, creator of the famous graham cracker, who promoted the importance of fiber in the diet and, in 1829, introduced the graham cracker. Today we accept, based on many studies, the benefits of high-fiber diets. Other fads, such as taking megadoses of vitamins or analyzing hair samples for subtle differences in trace minerals, produce only costly treatments for patients and small fortunes for those successfully promoting these approaches. They rest on little or no objective information about their benefits.

Special Nutritional Needs

What are the special needs of cancer patients? Obviously, if before cancer was diagnosed you had another condition that presented self-care challenges involving nutrition such as lactose intolerance, hypoglycemia, diabetes, food allergies, or underweight or overweight, the regulation and monitoring of your food intake remain important and complex. Beyond attending to these special needs, ideally you will follow the U.S. Department of Agriculture guidelines, including the famous food pyramid of fruits, grain, vegetables, etc., that should be consumed every day.

Maintaining weight is very important. Certain habits, such as eating three meals each day, are culturally defined but may not be appropriate for physiological needs. Indeed, for a cancer patient undergoing treatment eating four, five, or six small meals a day may be a more effective way to maintain maximum nutrition and caloric intake. Having slightly greater than your normal weight when entering into active treatment for cancer gives your body some extra storage of nutrients and an extra margin of error for those times when because of illness or its treatments you are less able to take in calories.

Treatments may negatively affect taste, smell, capacity to chew, even digestion of food. Such changes influence a person's visual and emotional reactions to food. When these changes occur, they need to be recognized and dealt with in a problem-solving fashion. Foods can be presented to make them more palatable from a visual, textural, and taste perspective. Sometimes foods are more palatable for individuals undergoing treatment when pureed or served either hot or cold. Familiar ways of spicing foods before illness may need to be altered to render them palatable after treatment. For some individuals the various forms of high-calorie nutritional supplement drinks or powders may become necessary. For a few, other forms of hyperalimentation or intravenous feeding of balanced nutrients, vitamins, salts, and minerals (TPN, total parenteral nutrition) may be essential. Utilizing such technologies aggressively has significantly enhanced the quality of life of many individuals and their capacities to respond to treatments, as well as lengthened life.

Be cautious about your use of alcohol, caffeine-containing drinks (including teas and soft drinks), and nicotine. Remember that these are all drugs in their own right, which when accumulated in the body can be quite toxic; they also affect the metabolism and hence blood levels and clinical activities of prescribed medications.

As we've said, your sense of taste and smell often change when you undergo chemotherapy or radiation therapy. This change may or may not be associated with a decreased interest in food and/or nausea. Often people are surprised to find that they are turned off to favorite foods such as coffee, tea, spices, slightly bitter salads or vegetables, and meats. Such foods in reality have more toxic products (bacteria, bacterial toxins, and heavy metals in small amounts) than other foods. While not much of a problem to a healthy person, it becomes one for someone with cancer and under active treatment. (No cancer patient under active treatment should eat raw seafood, particularly clams or oysters in any form. Even a mild shellfish-transmitted infection of viruses or bacteria can be enough to push a weakened biological system in the direction of further illness, further loss of function, or death.)

So, if something familiar is now repugnant, follow the wisdom of your body; it is simply trying to tell you that until you are healed you cannot handle that food. During the stressful time of active treatment, you are also more likely to develop sensitivities or outright allergic responses to proteins in foods that previously were not a problem. Common culprits are shellfish and mollusks, tree nuts, wheat, and eggs. Again, don't fret about such changes in your food preferences should they occur; simply admire your body's ability to guide you away from difficult-to-deal-with foods. Above all else, use common sense and do your best to maintain your weight.

Few physicians are trained in the nutritional sciences, but an increasing number are working with registered dietitians who do have such training. It really is a matter of common sense to think that the kind of fuel we take in—calories, vitamins, minerals—influences the capacity of our bodies to repair themselves, handle infections, and fight off the inappropriate and destructive changes caused by cancer. Educate yourself through the cancer diet books and recipes that can be obtained from the National Cancer Institute (1-800-4-CANCER) or your local branch of the American Cancer Society. Consult as needed with a registered dietitian who has the training and experience to deal with situations encountered by cancer patients.

Vitamins and Minerals

Recent research data on the positive effects of antioxidants have been impressive. Antioxidants help the cells of our bodies repair themselves. They seem to protect cells from chemical and radiation damage. Some minerals have antioxidant effects, but the safest currently known antioxidants are vitamins. Vitamin C and vitamin E are two widely used ones, and vitamin C is water-soluble, meaning that whatever the body does not need it eliminates easily.

Remember that vitamin A as an antioxidant in excessive amounts can be highly toxic, especially to the liver. Its precursor, beta-carotene, has not been shown by recent research to play a preventive role in cancers as had been hoped. Fat-soluble vitamins like A and E are an excellent example of the danger of common thinking that "if a little bit is good, more will be better." That is a dangerous way to think about any medication! Taking additional vitamin supplements with small amounts of trace minerals such as selenium, manganese, magnesium, and zinc may be a reasonable hedging of one's bets. Currently their safest form comes in standard brand multivitamins with trace minerals.

In late 1996 selenium received extensive publicity as possibly able to significantly reduce the occurrence of bowel, lung, and prostate cancer. Twice the usual daily supplement of one hundred micrograms was used in the study that generated all the publicity. But this was just *one* study, of only three hundred people. Once again, publicity outran science, probably causing a selenium ingestion fad. Selenium, like copper, cobalt, iodine, zinc, and molybdenum, can be poisonous to both animals and humans when taken in large amounts. Selenium can produce severe bowel irritability, chronic fatigue, and nerve damage. Indeed, excess selenium can result in death. So, before you take anything beyond what is found in over-the-counter vitamins with trace minerals, check with your oncologist, as well as with the National Cancer Institute and the Food and Drug Administration guidelines for safe levels of supplements. Taking some supplements may be unwise, even dangerous, with certain chemotherapeutic treatment regimens.

Sexuality

Sexuality does not refer specifically to genital sex, although that can be incorporated within it. It refers in the broader sense to our need to be touched and held and to our general responses to touching and holding. It reflects our origins, when we were contained and nourished within our mother's womb. Multiple studies of nonprimate warm-blooded animals since the 1950s as well as of humans have shown that without touch and holding infants do not thrive and frequently die. For example, there is a form of the wasting-away condition called *marasmus* (usually associated with protein intake deficiency) where human infants properly nourished and kept clean, but not nurtured through touching and holding, actually begin to lose developmental milestones, withdraw from human interaction, and, indeed, some die. As we grow, the effects of lack of touch are more subtle. Lack of touch does seem to undermine our body's energy flow and its capacity to maintain itself. This applies to everyone from older children to aged adults. Hence sexuality, as I define it, in its broader sense is an essential element of health maintenance.

Identify Your Needs

Each cancer patient needs to take an inventory of his or her own sexuality. What access to holding, touch, and, given your age, closeness with others and genital sex did you have before the diagnosis of cancer? You need to be frank with yourself as to whether there were preexisting unmet needs in any of those areas. Such unmet needs should be identified and addressed. Obviously touching and holding issues are of a different sort for a child with cancer versus an adolescent with cancer versus a young or middle-aged adult versus the elderly. The very basic issue, however, about the need for direct human contact and touch in some form is universal.

Sexual energies and even the interest others may have in providing any form of physical contact vary greatly based on a person's health status and attractiveness. *Attractiveness* refers, of course, not just to the physique but the kind of energy and spirit that an individual displays. If a person is in pain or overly fatigued, interest in any form of touch or sexuality is obviously reduced significantly. This does not necessarily mean that needs for at least the nurturance that occurs through touch is lessened. It may, indeed, be enhanced, but a person may be less able to seek or obtain such contact. Attractiveness to others for any form of interaction is also affected by how much anxiety the individual has and whether or not he or she is depressed. In addition, there are the specific effects of treatments. Sometimes these are the results of chemotherapy or radiation, which can render certain forms of touch, even all touch, painful. Fortunately, most of the time this unusual skin sensitivity is only temporary.

Self-Image and Sexuality

Other times effects of treatment significantly influence self-image. Some effects of treatment give all individuals a sense of altered self, even a sense of disfigurement. This may include loss of hair not only on the head but all over the body, changes in pigmentation, changes in body contours or indeed loss of body parts. Individuals, based on their cultural background, the community in which they live, and their own personalities, also vary greatly in how they are able to cope with these changes as well as the responses from others that may be desirable.

A seminar participant once spoke out about her complicated reaction to her surgery: "My husband seems very unconcerned about my changed appearance. I want to accept this as positive, but I would almost like for him to show some outrage at my scars."

Her mixed feelings not only quite correctly identified important concerns such as her anger at her disfigurement but also important and neglected limitations in communication between her husband and herself about their separate reactions to surgery.

Too often no one on your medical team asks about these changes. When they do ask, little is offered in assistance. I urge you to be aggressive on your own behalf in seeking assistance if you find you have any questions about either your sexuality or your sexual functioning. Your own physician may not have the knowledge or ability to be as helpful as you might need, but he or she certainly should be able to direct you to those who have the training to be of help.

"I've had a modified radical mastectomy with a saline implant. My husband of thirty-three years is impotent due to removal of the nerves during his radical prostate cancer surgery a year and a half ago. Now what? I am very athletic, healthy, and still feel a need for sex."

The woman asking this question did so in a Y-Me breast cancer support group meeting. What a sad statement about her health professionals that she waited for eighteen months before she found a setting that gave her the courage or permission to ask for help.

Coping with Changes

In terms of genital sex, it is important to be educated about the changes that can occur. For the male, chemotherapy can alter sexual desire and sexual energy and often can affect fertility. Fatigue and impaired energy because of chemotherapy or radiation therapy can create problems in erection and orgasm. Hormone therapy for cancer is being used more frequently in men, and it often alters sexual desire, creates erection problems, and always induces infertility. All of these problems can be modified with current medical knowledge. However, no one can help if the problems are kept a secret from the medical team. All too often the medical team forgets to, or simply doesn't, ask directly or give individual patients permission to ask questions about sexual functioning. Therefore such issues are never dealt with. (In informal surveys when I speak at large group meetings, I find that fewer than 10 percent of cancer patients indicate that their doctors have ever inquired about their sexual functioning.)

For the woman, chemotherapy can sometimes lower sexual desire, can often affect vaginal moisture, producing painful intercourse, and can often interfere with fertility. Certain forms of surgery and radiation affect sexual functioning, particularly when the surgery or radiation involves the pelvic organs. Desire may not be primarily affected, but often the capacities to respond with natural lubricants to sexual arousal are affected, creating painful intercourse.

Mastectomy and radiation to the breast, if they alter sexual desire at all, do so through a secondary psychological response to the changes and sense of disfigurement and perhaps to both verbal and nonverbal behavior of sexual partners. In no way does breast surgery or radiation directly alter the physiology of sexual responses. Some forms of hormone therapy in women, such as antiestrogen therapy, not only alter fertility but often alter sexual responsiveness in terms of lubrication when aroused, clitoral size and responsiveness, and sometimes sexual desire and the capacity of vaginal tissues to tolerate intercourse.

For both the male and female, some of the transient responses to chemotherapy, particularly in damage to rapidly dividing normal cells, produce conditions of inflammation of the mucous membrane that make sexual interactions unpleasant or painful. The healthy partners and spouses of cancer patients as well suffer from the pain, discomfort, even bleeding that they observe.

One seminar participant asked, "Do you have any suggestions for overcoming avoidance? That is, intercourse is uncomfortable physically and emotionally, so we avoid having it. That leads to guilt over avoidance, which leads to more problems with intercourse and more avoidance and more guilt."

The Essence of Sexuality

Nothing is more important than discussing human sexuality, and I use the term in its broadest sense—the touching, holding, and comfort that we all experience from birth onward from physical contact with others. For all people, though often in different ways, sexuality becomes anchored in physical sensations involving smell, taste, site, genital arousal, tension, and release, as well as being intimately related to self-image.

Sexuality and its expression in terms of touch are often diminished or even taken away from people when they are admitted to the hospital or are even diagnosed as having cancer. Friends and loved ones too often become distant. It is not infrequent, unfortunately, for cancer patients to have almost an "amputation" of sexuality by being deprived of touching and hugging, sensing less encouragement to continue their form of adult sexual expression, or even ordinary forms of physical interaction.

Family members become afraid to touch you. Doctors and nurses often give signals to friends and family that you have somehow become fragile, different, safe only to be related to cautiously and with distance. Yet touch remains essential to humans and to human health.

Research during the last twenty years on both mammals and humans indicates that touch, holding, and massage all produce positive changes that help move individuals chemically and physiologically out of the fight-or-flight mode into a relaxed state, one that allows healing. As a result, measurable increases in the activity of the immune system, particularly of the parts responsible for destroying unwanted visitors or unwanted new parts to our systems—such as cancer cells—occur.

As I noted earlier, studies that go back almost fifty years document how human infants, properly fed and cared for but not held, cuddled, or touched, can waste away and soon die from a disorder called *marasmus*. More recent studies have documented that premature babies when properly handled with touch and massage actually use both oxygen and glucose more efficiently and grow better. Even more recent studies indicate there is a decrease in depression in adolescents and adults as well as an improved sense of well-being with forty-five minutes of gentle massage twice a week. Thus touch, human contact, the normal laying on of hands, is essential to both health maintenance and to healing.

Doctors and Sex

Matters of adult sexual expression in good times are often difficult to discuss with your doctor. For cancer patients dealing with an oncologist it is often difficult for both doctor and patient. It should not be. Hopefully your oncologist will ask what your concerns are and suggest how you might maintain your normal level of sexual activity, seeking and reaching an appropriate and positive amount of sexual interaction and function for you. To help you in talking with your doctor, read the American Cancer Society's excellent booklets on sexuality for cancer patients. (See Appendix E.)

Are there additional reasons why adult sexual expression is so important? There certainly are.

Everyone faced with a serious illness feels disfigured and diminished, at least for a time. These feelings are increased by the experience of body changes—contours, pigmentation, scars from biopsies or more major surgeries or radiation, hair loss, fatigue, peripheral neuropathies, and weakness. Anxiety becomes a constant companion during the struggle to regain feelings of control. To adapt to and live with illness, you need to recapture diminished or lost functions and experiences. You also need to receive input from others that promotes hopefulness. Social and physical contact generates such hopefulness, restoring a lost sense of well-being, even of strength and energy.

Whether you are single, divorced, widowed, or married, seeking to recapture or approximate preillness levels of sexual expression helps with self-image and comfort. Sexual expression works (yes, even through chemical changes in the brain) against depression, helps contain anxiety, distracts from pain, improves sleep, provides a refuge from despair, and augments hope.

Focused Self-Advocacy

In 1992, a physician named Arthur W. Frank wrote, "Being ill is an activity for amateurs . . . most of us become ill without any particular training for the role. . . ." Many people discover that reason, willpower, and prayer—alone or together—do not carry them successfully through the odyssey of cancer. Other complex ingredients that we have been discussing thus far are essential.

Active involvement in the maintenance of your own health is one of these essential ingredients. The longer I practice medicine, the more respectful I become of the healing capacities of the human body. Wondrously complex, it continuously heals itself, replacing damaged subcellular and cellular structures, replacing whole cells, and completely renewing organ systems, such as skin and mucous membranes. Health maintenance involves accepting this reality while focusing your effort on giving your body a helping hand through enhancing its normal functioning.

Although you can improve your health by attending to the various issues discussed up to now in this chapter, do not become over-confident about your efforts before completing two other elements of the health maintenance inventory. These are assessing your vulnerabilities and examining your attitude and psychological state.

Assessing Your Vulnerabilities

All of us have vulnerabilities—areas of nonstrength. These often grow in importance even to the point of totally undermining us during periods of crisis. Identifying our vulnerabilities allows us to function as wise field commanders in a battle. We not only reconnoiter the nature of the enemy (the accurate diagnosis of cancer and the cancer type) and plan the attack (treatment decisions) with our technical experts (the oncologists) but also evaluate the weaknesses of our own side. That evaluation creates the potential for corrective action. Our goal is to strengthen our side and to be successful in battle.

In evaluating our vulnerabilities, we must think broadly as well as honestly. We need to ask ourselves about our physical and emotional selves, our family system, our constant preoccupations and concerns, our social and interpersonal skills, the known sources of extrafamilial support.

Focus, for example, on physical health. You may say "I have cancer. What else do I need to think about?" Well, life doesn't assure you that simply because it is threatened (and you with it) by the development of cancer you will not have other problems. Do not engage in denial or minimization: identify all problems you can. Be honest and thorough in identifying vulnerabilities to yourself. Among the common physical vulnerabilities are allergies, sensitivities to certain medications, overweight or underweight, hypertension, diabetes, chronic sinus infections, osteoporosis, gum inflammation, irritable bowel syndrome, hypo- or hyperthyroidism, migraine or tension headaches, and low back pain syndrome. There are many other possible conditions. The point is to identify those that exist and then do your best to control them, reducing the danger they may present to you as weak points in your total system.

Concerning nonphysical vulnerabilities, the same level of honesty with self is recommended and for the same reasons. Are you in a job you hate, in a marriage that makes you miserable? Are your children chronic problems? Are you dealing with any of this in an effective way? Is your educational background making for problems in communicating or in understanding medical issues of importance to you? Have you always been tentative and unsure of yourself, and is that now getting in the way of your becoming an active member of your own treatment team? Is a preillness awe or fear of people with special skills now interfering with your ability to relate to your doctors? Did you, before cancer, struggle to come to terms with your own aging and subtle decrease in abilities and energies in a way that fit with your memories but not your current condition? Is there anything you can do to make any of that better? Engaging in such an inventory is not an easy assignment in the best of times, and surely not now, but it is vital to your success in dealing with cancer and its symptoms.

What About Your Attitude?

The word *attitude* refers to your reactions to life experiences. It both reflects and colors your psychological state. Thus it may represent the most elementary item on the health enhancement inventory. Many people find themselves defining their lives in terms of their illness. Don't do that. Or, if you are already thinking and feeling that way, get help in escaping from a psychological trap capable of significantly diminishing your quality of life and possibly shortening life itself.

Our images of ourselves impact on our willingness to engage in the struggle for life. Physical appearance has significant importance. Dressing up, keeping yourself groomed and clean, is not merely done to please others. These activities also nurture you, helping you feel better about yourself. For this reason some years ago the American Cancer Society started its program for women called "Look better, feel better." That program tends to focus on dress, cosmetics, hair or wig styles. Over and over again it has been shown that individuals who participate in these programs have increased levels of energy, optimism, and hopefulness. Unfortunately, there is not yet an equivalent program for male cancer patients, despite the reality that the same coping principles apply to men.

All of us should monitor our moods, our body states, and our behavior. We need to ask ourselves if they are appropriate for the circumstances. We need to clarify our goals and reflect on them. We need to focus on the reality that most important among our goals is quality of life. We all need to put in the effort to define what that quality of life is. This too is a function of attitude and psychological state. The greatest challenge for many individuals is moving beyond anger and blame, both normal psychological reactions to a diagnosis of cancer. We need to resist thinking or behaving as we did in our younger years, when we wished to be taken care of by others in moments of crisis. We need to mobilize our resources so that we can cope when the reality is that we seek certainty when certainty is not possible.

Psychological State and Moods

And finally, it is very important to realize that cancer treatments themselves influence both attitude and psychological state. All treatments affect psychological states, whether it is the enforced healing after the surgery, the healing that is necessary when one has an infection, or the toxic fallouts of radiation or chemotherapy. Many physicians do not warn patients that all treatments influence psychological states on a transient basis. They tend to impair psychological functioning, emotional strength, and flexibility. Examples include the transient chronic fatigue that radiation can induce. Some chemotherapeutic agents can directly create problems psychologically, especially depression. So can the immunotherapies, some of which can produce not only depression but even psychosis.

Many chemotherapeutic agents can produce secondary physical effects that influence mood states, because they induce nausea and vomiting, weakness, the onset of pain, total body hair loss, or altered functioning of certain hormones such as thyroid and sex hormones. Understanding that changes in mood state may accompany treatments and are therefore transient and eventually manageable is key to health maintenance.

Distinguished former Rockefeller University research psychologist Neal Miller is quoted as stating, "The mind is the brain." Wrong! The mind is the brain *and* the body *and* the experiences of the individual in interaction with the environment throughout the individual's lifetime. The psychological self is a compound expression of everything within the individual as well as a constant influencing force on everything both within and around the individual.

Your psychological self and your attitude do influence your body's capacity to care for itself and to heal. It determines whether you ignore or are truly appreciative of, tuned in to, and respectful of your physical self. Use a positive attitude to do positive things for yourself. Use it to recognize and help you correct imbalances and problems when they occur, seeking the right kind of help. Use it to advocate for yourself with the medical system, your family, and, as needed, the community.

4

Taking Control of Pain: It's in Your Power

FOR MUCH OF OUR HISTORY doctors have been treated as secular gods who delivered their opinions without questions from their patients. That grew, in large part, from the patients' desire to believe in the healing skills, wisdom, and goodwill of their physicians. In exchange for promised positive changes in their health, patients endured whatever medicine or cure or procedure was recommended. Sometimes the treatment worked; sometimes it didn't. Either way, a kind of mystery surrounded anyone called *doctor*, and respect and honor came almost automatically with the title, whether education, talent, or skill commanded it. I don't describe the situation that way to belittle physicians but to clarify the base from which modern medicine has grown.

Until the 1950s Americans were not well-educated consumers of medical services. And the medical profession itself functioned with limited scientific knowledge compared to today. The second half of the twentieth century has fortunately seen an explosion of knowledge in all areas of science, including those related to health care. As a result the practice of medicine is infinitely more effective today than it was fifty, or even twenty, years ago.

We now know an immense amount more about the human body. The practice of medicine remains nonetheless a healing art as well as a science. It often performs incredibly well, but it is still accurately called an imperfect science. That's important to keep in mind.

While that old-fashioned tradition of unquestioned medical authority has eroded in recent years, it too often lives on as a remnant of yesterday. Even today most doctors speak to patients knowing (and expecting) that what they say will be accepted and unchallenged.

Catherine, after months of treatment with Prisolec for stomach ulcers, told her doctor that she had seen a television news story about the relationship between stomach ulcers and a particular bacterial infection. When she asked him to test her for the infection, he seemed displeased, but grudgingly did so. Her tests were positive, and she was started on an antibiotic. Her stomach pain disappeared. She stopped taking the Prisolec, and her doctor stopped being warm and friendly as he had been before. With his wrong diagnosis challenged, he became aloof and brusque. Catherine decided to find a new doctor.

You would think that getting to the truth would satisfy both parties. Unfortunately, it is not so. The unhappy reality is that too many doctors become defensive, irritated, and embarrassed when they are questioned or challenged by patients. You cannot let that stop you. Only you can redefine that timeworn relationship, that old broken-down health care hierarchy of one who directs and one who obeys. There is an alternative.

Be a Member of Your Treatment Team

The ideal doctor-patient relationship should be, as I have said earlier in this book, a collaborative one, not an authoritarian one. That is how American medicine should now be practiced and how it must be practiced in the future. Nowhere is this more important than in the treatment of chronic pain conditions. No one—not a doctor, not a friend, not a parent, sibling, or spouse—can fully understand or feel your pain. So it is vital that you make yourself part of your own treatment team. This will help you deal most effectively with pain.

All people with cancer experience at least some pain from procedures and tests. At least 35 percent experience treatment- or cancer-related pain requiring medication. Seventy-five percent of people with advanced cancer suffer significant disabling pain at some point in their illness. Fortunately, even if you suffer from chronic pain, you can be helped to handle your pain at a level that permits you to have a reasonable quality of life.

If a health professional ever minimizes your discomfort and your pain by implying or saying that it is "all in your mind," don't be defensive or feel hurt. Look that person in the eye and say that you agree because pain has to be in your mind for you to experience it. Pain, no matter where it originates, is always *in your mind.* If it is in your mind, then it is real: the mind and body are one. We'll return to this perspective shortly as we discuss pain.

Dealing with pain requires action on several fronts simultaneously:

1. You must be educated about pain as a phenomenon and about your pain in particular.
2. You must be able to understand, if not master, the psychological and behavioral techniques that have existed for ages for the management of pain.

3. You need to work to enhance your general health and well-being, using supportive techniques including ancient ones such as massage and gentle forms of exercise.
4. You should develop a treatment plan with your doctor, including a written flow chart of medications that can be used in handling your pain.
5. You should periodically review your treatment plan with your doctor.

All of this sounds as if it requires a lot of effort, and sometimes it does. But your efforts on your own behalf make a huge difference in how successful pain control is.

Understanding Pain

To help you understand pain, let's start by defining what it is not. It is not a disorder or a disease. It is vital to understand that. You may ask "If it isn't a disease or a disorder, what is it?" Pain is information, pure and simple. Pain is an attention-demanding, unpleasant alerting signal of varying intensity, quality, and rhythm that goes to your brain, indicating something is injured or not right, a something that may threaten your health or even your life.

Pain sets in motion changes throughout your body—size of pupils, heart rate, muscle tension, sweat gland activity, posture, immune system, and more. It also brings about changes in your feelings, thoughts, and actions.

Consider the simplest example. If you stub a toe, a message goes to your brain that the toe hurts, demanding that you should check for damage. Depending on what you see, you take some appropriate action. If it is serious—a deep cut or a fracture—you get help in dealing with it. If it is nothing more than a bad bump or a bruise, you wait for the ache to go away. You can't see the pain, but you can, in this instance, probably see the injury.

What if you didn't get the pain sensation when the stubbing happened? Some people with diabetes, for example, don't. They suffer from *peripheral neuropathy*, a condition in which the nerves that *should* carry pain signals do not. What happens to them under those toe-stubbing circumstances? If the skin on the toe were broken and there were no sensation of pain and nothing were done, infection might follow. Indeed, the infection might become so serious that it could lead to loss of the toe or toes, a foot, or even a leg.

So give pain its due. Essential for our survival in ordinary circumstances, pain helps us monitor our well-being and our healing. While it is hurtful, it can usually be helpful. At the very least, think of pain as information coming from an internal eye scanning your body. Think of it as a potential ally and friend in health maintenance and survival. This mind-set about pain may not make it any more pleasant, but it can make it more tolerable.

The Kinds of Pain

For you as a cancer patient, most pain is not as simple as a hurt toe. It is a serious message and needs to be monitored. You may experience pain that is *acute* (of short duration), *subacute* (of long duration but still transient), or *chronic* (never goes away). It may represent damaged tissue or injured nerves or a mixture of both. Acute and subacute pain are like that stubbed toe or the minor cuts and bumps and aches and pains we have all experienced in our lives—from the miseries of the flu or a fall or from a spurt of hot grease while cooking or a scrape while woodworking or from a twisted ankle when just walking. This kind of pain can last from minutes to many days. Acute pain, as when your vein is punctured to draw a blood sample, is very unpleasant but goes away within minutes or at least gradually decreases.

Chronic pain goes on for months or even years. It may be continuous, or it may be interrupted or change in its severity. The migraine headache condition is a good example of chronic but interrupted pain. If you have ever had one, you know how terrible it can be. It comes in varying degrees and only from time to time, but it does keep coming back.

Chronic pain does exist in less familiar and therefore more frightening forms than migraines. Particularly when chronic pain is connected with an underlying condition that cannot easily be healed, it becomes a significant impediment to quality of life. In such situations pain no longer serves a useful, self-protective purpose. It becomes like severe static on a radio—distracting and upsetting, making it difficult for you to listen carefully to what is being said, sung, or played. It becomes, unfortunately, useless—or certainly less valuable—information.

How Pain Is Perceived

In thinking about the experience of pain, it is important to know that pain is perceived differently by different people. You may remember from the playground when you were growing up that one child might fall and scrape a knee, get up without a whimper or with no more than a few tears, and be back playing almost immediately. Another child of the same age and the same sex and the same injury wept, sought out an adult for support or reassurance, and was immobilized for the rest of the play period. Which child were you? Those differences in response to pain are usually influenced by a combination of prior experience plus temperament. How you have learned to handle pain in the past defines, in large part, how you handle it later. You can learn, as one child did, to react with fewer tears and more immediately return to normal activities. It is not always easy, but it is possible.

As adults, you and I are creatures of our prior experience and temperaments, just like those children. Our pain, real as it is, is handled not only in terms of its immediate severity but also with reference to what we have learned about handling pain. We also react to the situations where the onset of pain has occurred—at home, in combat, in traffic accidents.

An early study of the influence of the circumstances of an injury on the experience of pain compared similar injuries in males of similar ages with how much morphine they requested for pain control. Those injured in combat during World War II requested significantly less than those injured in traffic accidents. In the war the injury meant you might survive and would be sent home. A traffic accident meant medical bills, loss of income, and other problems.

Pain's meaning and the suffering associated with it are further influenced by your health history, including emotional conditions and past painful experiences such as physical or sexual abuse, or preexisting conditions such as chronic anxiety or depression, disordered sleep, or disordered thought. Any of these can color the meanings of pain and your reactions to it, often without the treating health professional's awareness of such significant influencing factors unless you have made the effort to fully share the details of your life.

Pain in the Context of Cancer

When you are sick and experience pain but don't yet know what is wrong, you tolerate the discomfort by saying "People are caring for me, trying to find out what is wrong, trying to make me well." But that all changes when the diagnosis of cancer is made. From that moment on, any pain or new sensation from any source translates into fear of the unknown, fear of not being cured, fear of loss of control and recurrence, fear of death. Only when pain is experienced as a part of a procedure or treatment that you believe is necessary for potential healing or cure is it experienced with decreased fear and tension.

What you learn from health professionals at this point and how well you understand what you are told can greatly influence how you handle your fears. Just having questions answered, even when the answers are not what you would want, can help calm some fears by making the unknown known. Fears may continue and even grow at this time when both information and uncertainty contribute to a reduced sense of control. If you add to this feeling the nonverbal distress signals from health professionals and family—their anxiety, their restless projections of their frustration over not being able to help you feel better—your sensitivity to pain increases and tolerance of it decreases through the resulting greater focus on its presence.

Pain and its effects are also heavily influenced by other conditions. When your sleep has been difficult and disturbed, pain is always worse. When pain is associated with more than one place in your body or with physical loss or dysfunction involving the face, head, or neck, a breast, an eye, colon, or sex organs, powerful emotional reactions interact with and become part of the pain experience, creating a discordant symphony of discomfort and fear. When your pain is associated with weakness, loss of appetite or nausea, or changes in capacity to focus attention or think clearly, dealing with pain becomes very difficult. At best, you struggle to keep control.

Clarifying for yourself what your pain means to you can help you deal with the anxieties, fear, and depressed feelings that chronic pain generates in all who suffer from it. With the cancers, pain may be related to progression of your disease through growth of tumor in bone, internal organs, obstruction of internal organs, or growth on or into nerves and nerve roots. Pain may also be related to treatments: injured nerves postsurgery; gastrointestinal spasms; mouth, throat, esophageal, and rectal sores; sore muscles. Residual chronic pain can arise from radiation-induced scarring of nerve and other tissues or nerves disrupted to produce phantom limb or phantom breast pain or from obstructed lymph flow producing swelling of the involved tissues.

Finally, pain may also derive from noncancerous conditions such as arthritis and chronic low back pain syndrome. Your responses will be influenced as well by whether or not the pain is associated with moving about. Such clarification of your understanding can even help your family and friends. Their improved coping with your pain becomes a useful reinforcement for you as well. Any decrease in emotional discomfort decreases preoccupation with pain and encourages positive responses to pain treatments, freeing you up to focus on healing as well as on interests beyond your cancer.

Relating to the Experience of Pain

While pain has some universal characteristics, it has its own uniqueness for each individual. You cannot argue with it or disavow it. It is there, an unrelenting, undesirable companion. Reynolds Price described its constancy: "I was transfixed by the main sight in my view—my undiminished physical pain."

The experience of pain is described in many other ways as well. Those descriptions have important meanings to knowledgeable physicians and are an aid in helping them find the right combination of treatments, including medications, to make the pain more tolerable or even to eliminate it. Therefore, to help in your own care you need to focus periodically on examining your pain, just as you might examine a found object. Then describe to your physician how long you have had your pain and its characteristics. Let your doctor know how your pain is interfering with your abilities to carry out your normal activities and how that interference manifests itself. How severe is it? (See Appendix A for pain scales.) Does the pain affect your energy, your sleep, your ability to concentrate, your mood, your ability to read or calculate? What over-the-counter medications have you taken, if any? Have they helped? If they have helped, in what way? What other pain medications have worked for you in the past?

Describing Pain

We talk of pain as aching, itching or burning, like an electric shock, or sharp and stabbing, throbbing, dull, or intense. It may be localized, or it may involve several areas of the body. It may be felt as spreading from an original site to other places in the body. It may be simply a vague and diffuse feeling. It may be a new and unusual sensitivity of the skin to touch, cold, or warmth. Often, as with the stick of a needle, for instance, pain is acute and passes quickly. Sometimes there is lingering, decreasing pain that changes in sensation to throbbing soreness, aching, or tingling. Some of us feel pain as constant, some as cycling up and down in varying intensity with or without movement; sometimes pain comes in sudden bursts like lightning.

Pain, Fear, Tension

Pain, however it feels, however it comes and goes, is a negative sensory experience. The tolerance of pain, or your pain threshold, is unique. When that threshold is exceeded, different complicating emotional responses kick in. The emotion may be born of fear that damage has taken place to the body as a whole or to part of the body or to an internal organ. A pain/fear/tension cycle begins. Pain signals potential injury, making us vigilant and producing at least transient fear and concern. A few people may learn, depending on the nature of the pain and prior experience with pain, to easily overcome the initial fear. But for most of us pain leads to fear that cannot be ignored. Fear brings a focus, increased tension in reaction to the pain, and a preoccupation with all body functions and sensations, including an increased sensitivity to sounds and smells. Ever more alert to the pain and frightened, our ability to tolerate the pain diminishes further as the pain continues in duration and/or intensity beyond our expectations. Then, with this additional tension, there is an inevitable worsening of the pain. You find yourself on a downward plunging spiral.

Others in our immediate surroundings influence our reactions to pain. A doctor or nurse may grimace during a necessary but hurtful procedure. A family member or friend may react sympathetically toward pain, and that focus, concern, worry, and frustration out of a desire to help influences our responses and coping mechanisms. The reverse is also true: a confident, reassuring medical professional helps us get through procedures less traumatically. A calming, caring, reassuring friend or relative distracts us from our discomforts.

Pain's Impact on Self

With chronic pain you may feel broken, drained, demoralized, and diminished from how you remember yourself before pain became your constant companion. One patient described the experience as "a continuous siphoning off of my being." Another described it as making her feel "used up and thrown away." Others have used almost exactly the same words. More than one patient has told me, "It's like playing cards with half a deck."

You may feel a great isolation from others built on a dramatically increased self-involvement that never goes away. That mind state, in turn, unavoidable as it is, diminishes your capacity to be distracted by other things in life. Ironically, the capacity for distraction remains one of the consistently successful methods for coping with chronic pain.

Symptoms in chronic pain sufferers extend well beyond the pain sensations themselves. Symptoms include disturbing dreams, disruption of sleep patterns, irritability, guilt, and anger. They also often include decreased capacity to focus attention and to recall things known. You may experience decreased motivation, decreased interest in sexual activity, and even awake in the morning with the wish "Please God, take me today." This can add up to a dreary, drained-of-energy lifestyle, even clinical depression. (About 17 percent of people with chronic pain suffer from chronic depression in reaction to that pain.)

The fatigue and preoccupation with self produce a loss of spontaneity that in turn increases withdrawal from social interaction. Self-esteem diminishes. You may lose your job due to absences and/or poor productivity. A coworker or a health worker may whisper the accusation that painkillers have made you a substance abuser. If you are a patient who needs narcotics to function, chances are that your self-esteem will be further assaulted by dependence on physicians who are legally required to dole out your medications in relatively small amounts. You know that society may often confuse abusive use of drugs and your legitimate uses. You may even become aware that your doctor resists prescribing what you need for true comfort. Trust in doctors is frequently strained during these times.

Pain does make you feel trapped by your life and condition. You may find it hard to settle on priorities and to follow them when you do decide on a plan. You may remember how you acted in healthier times and try to perform just as you used to do, although altered capacities may make that both impossible and inappropriate. Time itself gets redefined as almost all things take longer than before you were ill. Self-care demands more time. Keeping a "stiff upper lip"—the too-easy advice of family and society—may suck up energies better expended on dealing with the reality of your pain.

With chronic pain you may observe yourself striving to present the appearance of normalcy to others. At the same time, when your determination to present a brave front works, you may find yourself resenting the responses you get. Instead of admiration for your efforts, you may hear comments such as "Well then, you can't be in all that much pain if you look so well and got here tonight!"

Engaging in Battle with Pain

Along with pain, dependency on others, as well as economic dependency on disability insurance payments and social programs, challenges your sense of worth. A final insult may come from disrespectful, humiliating, undiscerning comments that are offered gratuitously by some individuals that your pain can't be that bad—implying that it is made up or the result of an emotional problem.

All of this generates immense stresses. Dealing with it takes more energy from your already depleted energy supply. If you don't handle these stresses well, the resulting tension may make you focus even more on your pain and thus become more its captive.

Begin escaping from drowning in pain by refusing to battle with your personal reactions. Accept the legitimacy of the bursts of anger and resentment you feel. Accept as normal the feelings of guilt at being a burden to others as well as the fear, generated by changes in pain signals, that the cancer might be returning. Accept other unfocused fears.

Quality of life needs new defining; pleasures need to be rediscovered. All in all, an approach is required in which you adapt to modified expectations and learn to master life with chronic pain instead of feeling driven to be totally rid of the pain. Hope is redefined by seeing that even if you can't be "fixed," you can function and can strive (if you wish) for gradually increased functioning. You can redefine goals to experience even ordinary acts such as a completed load of laundry, a letter written, several telephone calls made—any one of these—as accomplishments.

Treatments

Remember that the experience of all forms of pain can be modified. A creative combination of treatments will almost always provide a reasonable quality of life. How is this *best* accomplished?

The answer begins with a partnership, a mutually respected collaboration, of patient and physician. This means that you and your doctor or pain team must think together about the symptoms you experience, tracking together how the pain symptoms are modified by medications and other medical treatment prescribed as well as by your emotional state, distractions, support systems, and work. We reach for this ideal approach of collaboration, recognizing that it is not yet the most usual form of care received by chronic pain patients. What follows are some perspectives on medications, psychological and behavioral approaches to pain management, self-care, and special pain treatment techniques. They are presented to encourage and empower you.

The Use of Medications

For health professionals and the public at large, medications of one sort or another understandably remain the focal point and main means of pain treatment. Healing herbs have been used by humans, as well as other higher primates, to help soothe pain and enhance healing since prerecorded history. More than six thousand medicinal herbs have been identified. They include popularly recognized ones such as aloe vera, the opium poppy, ginger, and two sources of aspirin—white willow bark and meadowsweet. Today, however, most of our medicines are laboratory creations. The application or ingestion of a medication is a very direct, visible, emotionally soothing, comforting response to the unpleasant or awful sensation of pain. Even though pain medications are sometimes overemphasized and often misunderstood, they remain the most common treatment in our society for pain associated with every ailment, including cancer. Used properly, they are an important ally for you.

Narcotics and Other Analgesics

All medications that reduce or eliminate pain are called *analgesics*. The opioid narcotics, originally derived from the resins of the poppy plant, form the most ancient class of medicines, other than alcohol, used to treat moderate to severe pain. Their use in pain management is much maligned. There is the belief in the Western world, particularly the United States, that they produce a severe secondary problem known as *addiction*. The popular image, at least one hundred years old, shows the opium-addicted person abandoning everything—family, job, health—in pursuit of "the pleasure of the poppy." It is true that addiction can result from the use of opium, heroin, and their narcotic derivatives.

Opium and heroin are not used for pain management in the United States. Derivative and synthetic narcotics are, however, widely used. The phenomenon of addiction is actually quite unusual for cancer patients and cancer survivors. Excellent studies show that individuals who take narcotics for a chronic pain condition rarely experience drug highs as are reported by people who use them for recreational purposes. It has also been found that cancer patients who have chronic pain rarely develop any kind of psychological dependence on the mood-altering effects of these drugs. The myth that narcotics are dangerous medicines for chronic pain is based on images of opium dens and heroin and morphine addicts created by Hollywood and cheap novels. In fact, for pain patients narcotics (with the exception of Demerol) may be safer than other medications used for pain. Tread carefully, but don't be confused by myths about drugs.

The opioids can with chronic use produce *tolerance,* which means that increased dosages of pain medications are needed to obtain the same pain-relieving results. This is often noticed first as the pain relief seems to be lasting for less and less time. There are many ways to prevent tolerance from happening if you work closely with your physician in monitoring and selecting medications and pay attention to the early warning sign of the pain relief lasting for a shorter period of time.

Opioids can produce physical dependence. This means that sudden cessation of the medicine results in withdrawal symptoms—sweating, chills, shaking, sugar craving, loss of energy, among others. Such symptoms are never life threatening, although they are frequently awfully uncomfortable. Concern about physical dependence should never keep you from the use of narcotics when they are useful and necessary. Withdrawal symptoms can be totally avoided with a measured, controlled reduction in the use of these medications once they are no longer needed.

Who gets adverse effects with narcotics and how strong these effects are varies from individual to individual based on how the individual absorbs and metabolizes the medicine, his or her level of illness, and the interaction of the opioid medications with other medications being taken. The most common adverse effect, constipation, can often be handled preventively by increasing water and fiber consumption. Adverse effects, besides constipation, include sedation, grogginess, dizziness, nausea, even vomiting. Respiratory depression, the slowing of the breathing control centers, can occur, particularly with the morphine-based drugs. (See Appendix A for commonly used narcotics and nonaddictive medications.) Other medications that provide analgesia by altering the activity of brain opioid receptors exist. They include a recently released nonaddicting medicine, tramadol, called Ultram.

The Nonsteroidal Analgesics

The most widely used group of pain-blocking medications is the nonsteroidal anti-inflammatory drugs. Many physicians include acetaminophen among these. That drug is widely marketed in the United States under various brand names, the most common being Tylenol. There are also many different forms of aspirin, also known as the *salicylates*.

The nonsalicylate anti-inflammatories (NSAIDs) range from such over-the-counter medications as Advil, Motrin, and Medipren (all three are actually the same medication, ibuprofen) to powerful newer substances that can be injected or taken as tablets such as Toradol (ketorolac). All of the nonsteroidal anti-inflammatory pain medications have adverse effects. Large amounts of acetaminophen can be toxic to the kidney and liver. It has been and must be used with caution by people who have problems with kidney and liver function (indeed overuse of this medication is currently the main cause of liver damage in Great Britain). The other nonsteroidal anti-inflammatories can, with chronic use, cause problems with blood clotting, stomach and intestinal bleeding, ulceration and even perforation, fluid retention, and swelling of extremities, and they may interfere with circulatory functions to the point of causing congestive heart failure. Addiction is unknown with these substances; tolerance is rare.

Adjuvant Pain Medications

There is another complex group of pain medications referred to as *adjuvant medications*. These medications make a huge difference in control of pain syndromes today. Many of them were originally developed to treat other conditions. They include the antihistamines, antianxiety agents, antidepressants, antiseizure medications, alpha and beta agonists, calcium channel blockers, muscle relaxants, neuroleptics, steroids, and stimulants. (These different general categories are outlined in Appendix A along with a table summarizing the front-line medications for pain.)

These medications do many useful things. Some help to quiet down irritable nerves; others decrease sensitivity to pain or, in other words, raise your pain threshold. Others reduce muscle spasm. Some reduce anxiety and tension. A few, acting as special stimulants to the brain, both counteract the sedative effects of narcotics and add to their potency, an effect called *synergy*. An even smaller number actually block the release of pain-inducing chemicals from the cells. Thoughtfully combined use of these medications constitutes some of the current art—as contrasted with science—of pain medication usage.

Six Rules for Medication Use

I offer six rules of proper use of pain medications for you to think about and discuss with your medical team.

1. Use pain medications in terms of specific target symptoms. That is, define and describe the location, characteristics, and severity of the pain (zero indicating virtually no pain, ten indicating excruciating pain). Also identify your reactions—anxiety, fear, fatigue, inability to think clearly, difficulty sleeping, depression, as well as muscle soreness and spasms. Different medications can target these different symptoms.
2. Treat early rather than late and treat when it is needed. Many people feel that it is important to be stoic, to handle pain without complaint as though it does not exist. I hope you don't. It is self-defeating and self-injurious to deny pain because you think you can gain respect that way from loved ones and caretakers. There is a balance between constant complaining and suffering in silence. Neither extreme merits a gold star. Pain must be treated as it is beginning to increase rather than when it is at its height. Treating pain when it is at its highest point requires much more medication and often results in a poor response. Pain should be treated on approximate schedules rather than a tightly prescribed three or four or six hours. You must listen to your body and take your medication at the beginning of an escalation of the pain.
3. Avoid confusion that can produce accidental underuse or overuse of medications. Even when you have a single medication to take, it is often easy to forget when you last took it, or whether you actually did take it, since other activities can well confuse you. There are many aids to help prevent such confusion. There are inexpensive plastic boxes with compartments labeled *A.M.*, *P.M.*, and

bedtime as well as with the days of the week. Lay out your pain and other medications in the different compartments in these boxes each week. An empty compartment means you have taken your medication. A box still filled when it shouldn't be tells you of forgotten doses. You must be careful: catching up is not the best way to deal with missed doses. In addition, if you have a prescription that permits you to take extra medication during the course of a night, never leave the entire bottle of medication at your bedside. In a sleepy state, you may take one or two and then not accurately recall in the morning what you did. Leave the bottle in another place. Don't put more than you need to take on a bedside table. Then in the morning you will know precisely how much medication you have taken.

4. Realize that medications for pain in today's world come in many different forms, and depending on your pain syndrome, your own physiology, and your own life rhythms, you should seek the one that best suits you. Sometimes pills work better, but more frequently medications in liquid forms are absorbed more rapidly and sometimes more efficiently. Various forms of injections exist. Medications may also be given as suppositories, through nasal inhalation, or in a form that you put under your tongue (sublingual). They may be worn as patches on the skin or received through infusion pumps to the bloodstream or spinal fluid.
5. Strive for functioning as fully as possible while containing and controlling your pain. Combine your pain medications and others you take in a way that preserves as much as possible the clarity of your thinking as well as your energy level. Accomplish this in the context of a pain-treatment plan that you develop and review periodically with your doctor.

6. Medications in combination often give a bigger bang for the buck than medications used singly. Also, since you will, as a cancer patient, most likely be taking medications for other reasons, the drug-to-drug interactions can be complex and almost always result in getting more of a response to a particular dose of pain medication than you would if you were not taking any other medications at all. Hence it is appropriate for you to start with low doses and work up to where you find appropriate pain relief.

Finally, remember that all pain and adjuvant medications are highly toxic when used in large amounts. Therefore, it serves you well to keep a complete list of all medications and dosages you are taking. Use only what your doctor prescribes, not more. Even in small amounts these medications can be very dangerous to children, so keep bottles out of reach of children in your household.

Psychological and Behavioral Approaches to Pain Management

The International Association for the Study of Pain defines pain as "an unpleasant sensory and emotional experience associated with actual or potential tissue damage." Clearly, psychological techniques—modifying thinking, feelings, and behavior *without* the use of medication—are essential to complete pain management.

These treatments include the different forms of group and individual psychotherapy, the behavior therapies, and hypnotherapy. All of these are too often considered mysterious processes. They are not magical; nor do you surrender control when you use them. They may produce astounding changes in behavior, feelings, and memory, yet none of them is beyond explanation and, indeed, they have many principles in common.

Distraction: A Universal Intervention

All of us have had some spontaneous experience with psychological and behavioral management. Parents, for example, always use distractions with children who experience pain. We attempt to involve the injured child, focusing attention on something other than the injured part and injured feelings. We comfort by holding, hugging, cuddling. We distract by making a face, a noise, nuzzling a child into giggles. We may offer a teddy bear or doll. As we grow older, having memories of being comforted when hurt, we learn to internalize our hurts and develop our own distraction techniques, including chores, work, writing, watching television, and listening to music to help ourselves. Distraction is, indeed, one of the basic psychological and behavioral techniques used by healers throughout time and the world.

Using Behavior, Feelings, and Thoughts to Cope

In practice, physicians frequently combine forms of all three therapies in various ways when helping pain patients. These therapies can be differentiated in terms of the following generalizations: the psychotherapies tend to focus on exploring, understanding, and modifying thinking styles and examining feelings and memories; the behavior therapies (with or without the technology of biofeedback) focus on understanding and modifying conscious as well as automatic behavior, particularly in response to specific conditions or situations (nausea when one sees the hospital or clinic where one had the chemotherapy); hypnotherapy uses the techniques of focusing attention with enhancing the universal capacity for distraction. (For example, you can train your mind to imagine yourself engaged in activity somewhere else during a lumbar puncture, thus distancing yourself from the pain and discomfort.)

In actual practice, when working with pain, expert physicians frequently combine all three therapies with patient and family education. Both the patient and close family members do best if they are taught about the particular form of pain suffered and about pain management and self-care in general. Your family should understand as well as it can the nature of the pain you feel and live with and be supportive of your pain control and health maintenance efforts.

Chronic pain groups can be very useful. They should have an experienced professional leader. A group environment gives you opportunities to vent your feelings to others free of the protective concerns you have when talking with family and friends. Groups also serve as places in which to share strategies and skills for coping with the pain.

The Psychotherapies

When the different forms of psychotherapies are used to help in chronic pain management, their goals are intended to give you a greater feeling of control. That includes a decreased sense of anxiety, tension, and depression and an increase in self-esteem and hopefulness. They should release more energy, moments of well-being, and the motivation to act, and they should decrease vigilance to pain signals. They should help pain become more like background noise rather than the major focus of your attention.

Describing these therapies as having characteristics of a professional art form captures the elements of them that go beyond what can be captured in textbook descriptions or flow charts. These elements tap into both the natural talents and experiences of the therapists and make the difference between mediocre and highly effective outcomes. Those natural talents and experiences incorporate capacities to interpret as well as understand unique dimensions of a patient's realities combined with a highly developed sense of the right time to present interpretations, launch behavioral changes, pace change processes, or solidify new approaches to dealing with pain.

For these reasons the experience and training of the professionals you work with is critically important to you. They must have credentials to assure you that they have been educated and have had a period of time of supervised clinical training. In addition, they should be able to present evidence that they have training and experience in working with chronic pain patients or at a minimum are currently being supervised by someone who has such experience. The professionals involved can be psychiatrists (they are physicians), anesthesiologists, internists, family physicians specializing in pain management, clinical psychologists, clinical social workers, or psychiatric nurse practitioners. Rarely do clerical counselors have such experience or knowledge. When properly conducted over a sufficient length of time (this length of time varies with each situation but on the average involves about twelve months), the contributions that can be made to the chronic pain patient's quality of life are impressive. (Do remember that only the physicians and nurse practitioners have the training to interpret the influences of medication.)

Whether you are in individual or group therapy, you should be able to examine and understand fears that you have associated with pain and discuss and describe the dimensions of the pain experience. When you put the pain in that context, it helps you feel more in control. You can work on changing the way you describe your experiences to yourself, working toward decreasing negative thinking and overgeneralizing about pain experiences. This will help keep you from making more out of bad situations than already exists.

Hypnosis and Hypnotherapy

With hypnotherapies you can combine relaxation and slow deep breathing techniques to set a stage in which you imagine yourself in a safe and comfortable place other than where you are. Once you have captured with all your senses in your imagination being in such a place, you should be able to examine your pain and describe it in terms that give the pain a shape and color and other characteristics you may attribute to it. At that point you may be asked to see if you can diminish the pain, particularly in terms of its size and the intensity or the color of the pain. Sometimes this is done by suggesting to you that you may want to look at the pain as you might look at an object when turning a pair of binoculars around the wrong way, therefore making what you see through the binoculars much more distant. Sometimes hypnotic suggestion focuses on transforming the pain into another feeling, place, or even throwing it away.

Other hypnotic techniques involve creation of dials on machines that you can turn up and down with associated gauges indicating a lessening or enhancement of pain or focusing on feelings of numbness from cold or a Novocain type of anesthetic. Hypnotic techniques can work very well as long as the individual is not in an unusual state of anxiety or in a state of severe, escalating pain.

Behavioral techniques include various forms of relaxation as well as specific ritualized exercises for changing unwanted thoughts. They also include biofeedback, which was described earlier. Again, biofeedback electrodes attached to different areas of the skin read muscle tension, peripheral temperature, and sweat gland activity. You may be trained to visualize images and sounds, allowing you to reduce muscle tension and enhance functioning of other areas of your body. Through such techniques you can learn to recognize and understand signals from your body. You can determine which sensations you should be concerned about as potential or possible warning signs to be rechecked periodically, which sensations can be ignored, as well as which sensations represent signs of healing. The capacity to turn down at will, as in a rheostat, or eliminate the alerting and fight-or-flight response that is associated with the tension of the experience of pain can add significantly to your capacity to live with chronic pain.

Health Enhancement in Pain Management

Managing your general health is essential to proper management of chronic pain. This means that you should strive for correction of any problems of sleep, improvement of energy flow throughout the body, a balanced musculoskeletal system, optimal nutrition, and maximum use of family and friendship resources for emotional and practical support. Chronic sleep deprivation produces irritability and the symptoms of depression—loss of motivation, decreased energy, negative thinking, and anxiety.

Sleep Management Is Essential to Pain Management

If you suffer from chronic pain, you must inform your physician about what your sleep cycle was before there was any illness or pain and what the normal sleep cycle in the family was. You should be aware that sleep is something that should come naturally after not more than twenty minutes on most occasions. If the length of time it takes to fall asleep goes much beyond that, we speak of it as being a *sleep latency* problem. This is one of the very common problems that individuals with chronic pain have that begins a cycle of disrupted sleep with all its consequences. Not infrequently medication may be needed to help with the sleep cycle. Such medications do not have to be addicting. In addition, there are behavioral techniques using relaxation exercises that can help individuals without medications to improve their sleep cycles. Finally, in terms of sleep, it is important to focus on sleep hygiene. Sleep hygiene refers to having good habits including going through a period of natural distraction before bed—gentle stretching, warm baths or showers that help signal the body that it is a time for "letting go" and decreased vigilance.

Another important dimension of sleep hygiene is to avoid the use of television or movies in the hour before you wish to fall asleep. Both of those media are designed to be highly stimulating to the central nervous system, and though they provide companionship and distraction, they work against the necessary processes that allow an individual to naturally fall asleep. Sleep medications should be the last line of defense but may be necessary. They fall into the categories of herbal, over-the-counter, and prescription medicines. When required, they too are among the adjuvant pain management medications. Some of them are reviewed in Appendix A.

Exercise and Pain

Healthy body balance must be striven for in the context of chronic pain or any chronic health problems. Regular exercise at a level that the individual can tolerate is helpful. Such exercise includes walking as well as the gentle movements that are available through the oriental exercises of tai chi or qi gong. These all represent repetitive exercises that can be done even by individuals who are confined to sitting up in bed or in wheelchairs, providing some level of aerobic conditioning.

All such conditioning exercises take time. Our culture is an impatient one, and people want quick results. Toning of the body and facilitating healthy energy flow cannot be accomplished instantly, on command, quickly. But given time, positive results can reliably be expected.

Often chronic pain patients should see a physical therapist in consultation. Most important in terms of body balance is the physical therapist's identifying areas of guarding postures, modified postures that a person assumes to help him or her feel immediately more comfortable with the pain. These modified postures often result in secondary muscle spasms and injuries to the ligaments, tendons, and the coverings of muscles, with a worsening of the pain syndrome. Appropriate stretching and strengthening exercises can be taught by a registered physical therapist. In instances of significant weakness or fatigue such exercises need often be conducted in a situation of reduced gravity. This is best done by exercising in a swimming pool of mild temperature.

Massage and Pain

The ancient techniques of massage are also helpful to energy flow and balance. Massage may include use of local hot or cold compresses, vibration, tapping, or pressure. The healing touch in massage has been used in many cultures throughout recorded history to aid in general well-being. Recent research does demonstrate that massage has positive effects on our sense of well-being and how we mobilize our healing capacities.

Nutrition, Caffeine, and Alcohol

Nutrition, as has been discussed in earlier chapters, is critical to body health and balance, but especially so in pain patients. Pain patients must do their best to maintain their nutrition as well as make use of available nutritional supplements based on current knowledge. These nutritional supplements can include not only vitamins and the subcategories of vitamins called *antioxidants* but also mineral supplements such as selenium, magnesium, and calcium. Review of your standard intake of substances is important, particularly when you usually pay little attention to caffeine. Caffeine may be very helpful in the management of pain, but excessive amounts of it may produce irritability and overreaction to unpleasant stimuli.

Finally, many physicians and their patients forget to look at the issue of alcohol and its use by chronic pain patients. We all know it as perhaps the original pain-relieving substance. However, alcohol in large amounts is a neurotoxin; that means that it can injure peripheral nerves as well as the brain. On a short-term basis it can serve to distract an individual with pain and numb responses to pain. Alcohol is not an effective pain medication for chronic use. Indeed, one of the causes of nonresponsiveness of pain patients to pain medications and to treatments such as acupuncture is unrevealed chronic use of alcohol or alcohol dependence. Alcohol-dependent individuals absorb and metabolize medications very differently from non-alcohol-dependent people. It is most important in helping yourself with pain that you be honest with yourself as well as with your physicians about your use of alcohol. Especially when pain derives from damaged nerves, alcohol may intensify it.

Electrical, Mechanical, and Invasive Techniques in Pain Management

A very popular form of pain management over the last twenty years has been transcutaneous neurostimulation, or TENS. Tiny electrical currents of low voltage and low amperage are delivered by a device in a cyclic, pulsating fashion. TENS has been found to help some individuals with pain. TENS units are approved by the FDA as medical devices. There is some controversy based on prospective research studies concerning their true usefulness, however. One explanation about how they may help is called the gating theory. It hypothesizes that the electrical stimulation through the peripheral nerves to the spinal cord blocks pain signals as they are sent from the spinal cord to the brain.

Another theory suggests that the TENS unit's electrical stimulation forces the body to produce more of the natural pain-relieving substances called *endorphins* than it usually would produce, resulting in a decrease in pain perception by the individual. A third theory refers to the TENS devices as doing both simultaneously. Finally, there is a belief that TENS devices have no significant effects on the pain itself other than the electrical stimulation's providing a source of distraction from the pain.

Various forms of electrical stimulation devices are now being experimented with in certain medical centers around the country where the electrical stimulation is applied to nerve routes or directly in spinal cord stimulation. Again, such uses are considered experimental. In my opinion, TENS devices have very limited effectiveness despite the fact that they are still readily approved by many insurance companies.

Acupuncture

Much better documented are the effects of acupuncture. As of 1996, acupuncture needles were finally approved as legitimate medical instruments for control of pain and nausea by the Food and Drug Administration. Not only is acupuncture believed to help the body energies flow better, but it has been documented to specifically release endorphins from the brain or increase production of these natural pain-relieving substances. Acupuncture needles after placement may also have electrical stimulation added to them. All acupuncturists in the United States today use sterile disposable steel needles. These are now required because of the threat of both AIDS and hepatitis.

The effects of acupuncture seem to be cumulative. Almost all individuals who expect to have one or two acupuncture treatments to relieve pain will meet with disappointment. In my experience you are looking at a series of at least ten to twelve such treatments before you can evaluate if they are providing relief from pain and producing additional salutary effects. If you see an acupuncturist, verify that he or she is licensed by your local medical society or state government.

Invasive Analgesia Techniques

Other invasive ways of dealing with pain include techniques that have become the area of expertise of specifically highly trained anesthesiologists. Indeed, pain management has become a subspecialty within the specialty of anesthesiology in the United States. These anesthesiologists work mostly by injecting various anesthetic and inflammation-reducing agents into the body in specific areas. These injections are referred to as *trigger point injections* and *nerve blocks*. In special situations substances are injected that actually can destroy nerve functioning on a temporary or even permanent basis. For those individuals who might be candidates for this type of pain treatment, I encourage you to make sure the physician in question has been certified as a pain specialist by the American Board of Anesthesiology.

Anesthesiologists today work with general and neurosurgeons to implant catheters that can administer narcotics into the cerebrospinal fluid for pain relief. The metering out of pain medication can be computer and patient controlled. Electrical spinal cord stimulators are also being tried at some treatment centers. Careful evaluation and thoughtful consent are needed for all these procedures.

Finally, there are certain surgical techniques reserved for the terminally ill who have not received relief from any of the other forms of pain treatment. These techniques involve the cutting or destroying of peripheral nerves. There are even some neurosurgical forms of these techniques that involve sectioning of parts of the spinal cord roots, parts of the spinal cord itself, or sectioning pain receptors within the brain. I question the value of those techniques. First, the body has immense capacities for healing itself and has multiple duplicate pathways for giving and receiving signals. As a result one may destroy one pathway, only to have another one assume the same responsibilities, resulting in a return of some form of pain. Second, the surgical and brain tissue destroying techniques are really quite primitive as a way to deal with the problem of severe pain. They presume that simply by cutting or interrupting the hard-wiring of one part of our system we can diminish pain perception.

What we have found, unfortunately, is that individuals in whom those techniques have been used and who are not terminally ill, or live more than six months, often go on to develop worse sensory experiences. These include very unusual forms of pain and temperature perception, phantom pains, and intense unpleasant feelings of numbness that produce very high levels of anxiety and even disorientation. We have found that the interruption of pain fibers and permanent destruction create only a very transient relief of pain and tremendous disappointment and a secondary depression. Finally, for such individuals who have submitted themselves to these techniques, the pain sometimes returns at even higher levels than before.

A single intervention never "fixes" pain. Chronic pain in particular must be treated with a thoughtful combination of treatments. These include education of patient and family, thoughtful use of medications, proper self-care, and mind-body regulation interventions. Sometimes highly specialized techniques may be required. Above all, please remember that a great many things exist to reduce suffering.

5 Nontraditional Treatments: The Choice Is Yours

CANCER, AS YOU KNOW too well, complicates your life in many ways. One complication comes in having to make difficult choices about treatment when you never feel you know enough about all the options. It is tough enough with traditional choices: chemotherapy, radiation, surgery, or some combination of them. But choices don't end there, and sometimes they don't begin there either.

You may have a cancer that is so slow in developing that no treatment is recommended. Or you may be in remission. Just waiting without doing anything may seem intolerable to you. It is even worse if your doctor says there is no additional treatment he or she recommends.

Barbara, a fifty-four-year-old professional, noticed a hard lump where her breast extended to her left armpit. She sought immediate medical consultation, obviously fearing a diagnosis of breast cancer. The biopsy of a lymph node revealed that she had a form of lymphoma. After all the tests were complete, she was told that the cell type and extent of her cancer indicated a very slow-developing form. The recommendations were to watch and wait, to receive no treatment until the disease became more active. Second and third opinions at world-class cancer treatment centers were the same: be closely observed by your doctors, but undertake no treatment now. Barbara was frantic. "I have cancer. How can I live with no treatment? I've got to do something."

It was overwhelming and confusing. How could she decide what to do? In response to her call for help and hope, her husband, family, and friends started a barrage of suggestions about alternative treatment. She wanted to fight her cancer and to improve her health, not just sit and wait to get sicker.

Barbara's wish drove her, perhaps like you and some of your friends, to learning about alternative or nontraditional treatments outside the mainstream of traditional Western medicine. Currently many physicians greet the idea of these treatments with suspicion if not derision. Both reactions are based in part on lack of knowledge and training beyond the walls of Western medicine. Gradually this situation is changing, even in the curricula of some medical schools. (About a quarter of them now offer at least one course in alternative medicine.) If you are fortunate, you will have doctors whose knowledge helps you navigate a complex world of nontraditional as well as traditional therapeutics and other remedies without harm to you or to your pocketbook.

Common Sense, Hope, and Illusions

Hope is a vital part of your desire for a cure, but you need to keep in mind that this is also a time when wishes untempered by common sense, hard questions, and careful reflection can, at great emotional and financial cost, make a bad decision worse and make you a victim all over again. Hope based on what is real is valuable; hope based on illusion is not.

In those moments and days after you have accepted the diagnosis of cancer, even once you have begun treatment, a surge of disbelief may roll over you. "Do I really have cancer?" As you listen to your doctor, you may in your desperation hear promises that were not given, or you may fail to question the doctors adequately about the future. Your mind is clouded by your fears, anxiety, confusion.

Even once you have accepted the diagnosis of cancer, even once you find yourself participating in treatments and follow-up care, you experience flashes of disbelief. You notice moments during which you find yourself bargaining with some power outside yourself and wishing for things to improve, for a good outcome.

While wishing doesn't always make it so, dreaming of perfect health is hard to avoid. It is a time when you may listen to promises of better health and possible cure delivered by nontraditional healers. Friends, family members, and interested acquaintances have reactions similar to yours. Through their intense desire for you to find good health and achieve a cure, they are especially open to the claims of all sorts, often as trumpeted by stories in the media as well as by clever, sometimes deceptive, marketing. (In 1996 American consumers, almost exclusively out of their own pockets, made nontraditional medicine a $14 billion industry! Money well spent? That is not clear.)

Frequently friends and relatives bring articles to your attention about new treatments—some may be new drugs, others nontraditional treatments. They may even aggressively insist, against your own inclination, that you investigate a new treatment they have heard about at work, seen in a magazine or tabloid, found on the Internet. Sometimes their well-meaning involvement does transmit helpful information. Often, however, their advocacy is simply confusing, adding pressure and therefore more stress to your already stressed existence.

How Do You Guide Yourself?

Certainly nontraditional systems contain insights worthy of study and of use. Over the last ten years leaders in traditional medicine, including the National Institutes of Health, have become more and more open to examining many unfamilar forms of health maintenance and healing found scattered throughout the world. So, during this time of increasing openness to other forms of healing—and we are just in the early phase of such change—how do you guide yourself?

Combine common sense with a heavy dose of clear thinking. Understand what makes traditional Western medicine different from nontraditional treatments. (See the next section.) Test what you hear. Figure out what your wishes are and what really is being offered. Ask yourself if you are hearing only anecdotes, promises, and personal testimonials, not substantiated facts. Only then can you be sure to avoid becoming a victim of individuals and systems that prey on your wishes to be free of illness.

Bear in mind that there is a long history of people peddling miracle treatments that don't work and that the tradition continues and thrives today, energized by our entrepeneurial spirit. When that hard sell combines with the powerful wish to find simple answers for even complex health problems, a dangerous mixture results. It may place you at risk for loss of time, loss of money, loss of improved health, even loss of life!

Combine Common Sense with Openness to Change

A commonsense starting point is reminding yourself that if any nontraditional system of medical practice from Ayurvedic medicine to herbalism to homeopathy had a corner on the market of wisdom, health, healing, and longevity, it would have become the predominant health care system in the world a long time ago.

None of them has achieved that status. But they all have their niches; some are helpful and, as a result, have begun to influence or are considered complementary to many forms of traditional medicine. Old ideas about nutrition are being reexamined, ancient herbal medicines studied, and ancient techniques have been embraced over the last ten years. For example, as of March 1996, the U.S. Food and Drug Administration (FDA) classified acupuncture needles as legitimate medical instruments, completely opening the door of Western medicine to this ancient approach to health maintenance and healing.

Biofeedback also finds itself more and more in the mainstream of modern medicine, as do massage, nutrition, and the immunotherapies. As I write this, the world of healing moves toward a greater and greater openness of mind and spirit, which will eventually profit all of us, yielding a thoughtful integration of the traditional and nontraditional. This is just a beginning.

Separating Traditional Medicine from Nontraditional Medicine

Traditional Western medicine and surgery are supposed to be based on systematic observations, thought, and study over meaningful periods of time that result in treatments that produce measurable and repeatable positive improvements in function and in health. Once effectiveness has been demonstrated, any competently trained, responsible person should be able to replicate the surgery or treatment if given access to the same resources and should be able to obtain positive results more than 50 percent of the time.

This process of observation, thought, and study allowed what were once nontraditional or outrageously daring ideas to become basic elements of modern health care: the germ theory of disease; immunization; sanitation systems for water and waste; anesthesia for surgery; blood transfusion; extracts of botanical sources to produce dramatically successful medicines; mineral sources to treat illnesses; radiation as treatment; chemotherapy; substances to alter the functioning of bacteria, fungi, and viruses; staples to close wounds; major surgery performed without cutting open a person; genetically engineered substances to help the recovery of red and white blood cells.

Nontraditional systems of health and healing have not measured the outcome of their work as our traditional medicine does. (This has proven particularly dangerous with herbal medicine. See Appendix B.) Many of the nontraditional systems rely significantly on the charisma of the practitioner and the length and quality of time spent with the patient. Time spent and charisma are important, but they are not major concerns of our traditional biomedical approaches to care.

Alternative Treatments

An examination of alternative medicine reminds us that mankind has struggled for centuries to improve health and reduce suffering. Some techniques such as drilling holes in the skull to cure severe chronic headaches provide frightening reminders of how desperate both patients and healers can become in their search to obtain and provide relief. Others such as the case of severe brain and nerve damage from mercury-tainted dolomite (a calcium source) or poisoning from potions of bloodroot and mahuang (*Ephedra sinica*) remind us being called *natural* or having its praises sung by others does not make a substance safe or good.

Many of the alternative treatments provide some comfort without harm. Some treat certain conditions other than cancers quite well. They can be useful because cancer patients can obviously have, in addition to their cancer, other health-related problems. In addition, some help reestablish a sense of well-being.

Seeking ways to mobilize nature's healing force drives the interest we all should have in healing. Many nontraditional methods are used in the context of healing rituals that remind us that the "foot bone is connected to . . . the head bone . . . and they all have to walk around." By this I mean that such rituals suggest the importance of putting our efforts into rebalancing and regaining health for our entire body, not just into trying to corral and eliminate the cancer cells.

Often when people talk of alternative medicine, they cite the occurrence of spontaneous remissions or regressions in cancer. They certainly do happen, but they do not occur as a predictable phenomenon with any one form of alternative medicine treatment any more than they do with Western medicine (surgery, chemotherapy, or radiation). Spontaneous remissions, by definition, occur in response to unknown factors or events.

I have often seen nontraditional treatments be useful to patients. I have *never* seen a cure or a miracle in response to one of them. Please just remember at least that when you bargain or pray for hope, you are most vulnerable. It is true that nontraditional and alternative treatments are moving into the mainstream. (So again are the practice of religion and the use of prayer.) But be cautious of fads and the normal wishes we all have for magic.

Use nontraditional therapies if you wish, but as complementary treatments when your cancer is not in remission, never instead of known, established treatments. After your remission, use those that comfort you and help you in the challenge of living with your uncertainties. Make sure that the alternative treatment does not hurt you physically and does not hurt your pocketbook.

My clustering of nontraditional and alternative practices (referred to by some as *complementary healing*) derives from an approach to the subject developed by the Office of Alternative Medicine of the National Institutes of Health. Definitions are, of course, with reference to the standard medical system in the United States at this time. There are five different nontraditional fields of practice: (1) alternative professionalized systems of health practice (traditional oriental medicine, Ayurvedic medicine, homeopathy, etc.); (2) adjunctive forms of health maintenance and healing (mind-body interventions, diet and nutrition, manual healing methods); (3) bioelectromagnetics; (4) pharmacologic and biologic treatments; (5) herbal medicine.

Those nontraditional practices most comfortable for me represent approaches to healing and well-being used for thousands of years by millions of people who can't all be deluded. These practices, when applied by properly trained practitioners, comfortably fit with the Hippocratic oath to "do no harm." They consist of acupuncture; the manual healing methods, particularly massage; and the mind-body techniques, including biofeedback, relaxation, hypnosis, and guided imagery. Since I have written earlier about mind-body techniques, I will describe briefly here what I know about acupuncture and manual healing. A broader review of alternative treatment approaches is in Appendix B.

Acupuncture

About two thousand years ago or more, a sharp stone tool was used to lance infections. By A.D. 618 the procedure had evolved into the use of sharp metal needles to treat illnesses, and the process was taught at the Imperial Medical College in China. What we now know as acupuncture, in both the East and West, still involves metal needles, but today once in place their effects may be enhanced by either manual or electrical stimulation.

Acupuncture was first practiced in the United States in the late 1800s, but it was not until 1996 that the FDA declared that acupuncture needles were legitimate and safe medical devices. Today's needles are made of disposable stainless steel and vary in size and length, but the largest (about the width of a human hair) is half as wide as the finest intradermal syringe needle used today. Its tip is sharp, having no cutting edge. The techniques of insertion, needle size, and depth vary from acupoint to acupoint.

What we know today is that acupuncture releases various natural chemicals called *endorphins* that are associated with pain and temperature and immune system modulation. There is definitely a neurochemical, neuroelectrical, and neurophysiologic basis for acupuncture.

With acupuncture, specific sites on the skin are stimulated. These sites, or acupoints, are way stations for the body's vital force. They have high electrical conductance and are often associated with increased blood circulation.

Skin around an acupuncture point may become slightly reddened, warm, and raised, but not nearly as much as from a mosquito bite. Many people feel a sense of tingling, expanding fullness, and spreading warmth around the needle site. There is rarely any sensation of pain or important discomfort. Most people feel relaxed, even sedated, over the course of an individual treatment. After treatments and a brief rest period, others are energized, even euphoric.

About a quarter of patients endure minor side effects: discomfort or small areas of soreness or small black and blue marks from the needling, light-headedness, clammy skin, queasiness. The last three side effects often are avoided if the patient lies quietly for twenty to thirty minutes after a treatment is completed.

A series of treatments usually runs for six to ten weeks, often starting with two or three treatments a week and then diminishing; if after no more than fifteen treatments no positive changes occur, the treatment should be stopped.

Manual Healing Methods

These healing methods may be the most ancient of all. They are all based on the use of touch with fingers and hands; thus they all appeal to our earliest origins and the meeting of our earliest needs to be held, touched, and thus comforted. All of these methods—some very widely used in the United States—have in common the belief that any discrete body part often affects secondarily the function of other discrete, not necessarily connected, body parts, even those at a distance. All methods work toward creating harmonious balances within the individual. Different methods manipulate soft tissues, and some attempt to realign body parts, claiming that these realignments and manipulations restore neuromuscular function and improve visceral organ health. All manual methods, when used appropriately and administered properly, can help an individual feel better. They can help a person feel more relaxed, feel relief from muscular and tendon soreness, feel nurtured, experience improved energy, feel comforted and reassured. Evidence exists that some of these techniques do transiently improve immune system functioning.

Massage Therapies

There are at least eighty different defined methods of massage therapy. All are based on manipulation of soft tissue only. In various forms they seem to have been practiced for thousands of years in the Far East, in Persia, Ancient Greece and Rome, medieval Europe, and, of course, today. Their purpose is to encourage the ability of the body to heal itself. Nineteen state governments, at last count, license massage therapists. Their national organization, the American Massage Therapy Association, has more than twenty thousand members.

All massage therapies manipulate the soft tissues of the body for the purpose of reducing muscle spasm and tension, improving range of motion, and improving the interactions of the different components of the soft tissues including fascia, blood flow, and lymphatic drainage. Some techniques emphasize using pressure points and are therefore similar to acupressure; others focus on modification of posture; some are very aggressive, even painful to experience, while others are gentle and soothing. Many combine the different approaches.

The names of some may be familiar to you: Swedish massage; deep tissue massage; Rolfing; manual lymph drainage massage; shiatsu; tsubo; Alexander techniques; Feldenkrais; bioenergetics. All techniques have their avid adherents, their devoted followers. All when practiced by competent, experienced, and responsible individuals can comfort, relieve symptoms, and help people cope with a chronic illness. All present an additional demand for out-of-pocket expenditures. I do recommend combinations of the gentler techniques, postural work, and trigger point work to those who can afford these services.

6 Family and Friends: They Make a Difference

WHEN YOU HEAR the diagnosis of cancer, you inevitably think first of yourself. It is, after all, your life that is at risk, your burden to carry, your lifestyle that will change. To be anxious, filled with stress and anger, and even to be depressed is normal. At the moment of diagnosis you may feel stunned, unbelieving, terribly alone with constantly shifting thoughts and fears.

But you must remember at a time like this that you are not alone. Most of us are part of a family or friendship network. Your success in dealing with your cancer may well depend on how well your family also deals with it. This may seem odd to say, but it is true. If family members do not handle the situation well, they cannot provide the support you will need. Don't exclude them.

For all members of the family, life, although not defined in terms of your cancer, must be defined with reference to it. It is a difficult time to keep things in balance. There are many places where you and they can stumble. When that occurs, all of you will find yourselves at high risk of becoming victims of the fallout of the disease and its treatments, with the quality of your life, and perhaps theirs, diminished.

What all of this means is simple: *Cancer is a family disease*, not genetically speaking but in its impact. Make no mistake about it. When the disease strikes one person, it affects many. When cancer is diagnosed in one family member, it touches the entire family, including the healthy ones.

As a cancer patient, you may not always have the patience or even want to take the time to understand how your illness affects those who care about you and love you. But it is important, really vital, that you understand that an emotional burden spreads quickly and inevitably to those who are close. It even shows up in physical ways. There is no question that family members of a person with cancer, after the diagnosis, suffer more illness, need more doctoring, use increased amounts of health resources, and not just briefly but for extended periods.

Their problems—anxiety, headaches, chronic lower backaches, intestinal or sleep problems—may seem minor compared to your cancer, but the misery those pains cause is real, it results in endless distress for them, and it diminishes the quality of support you need.

Janet, fifty-four, recently learned that her husband had cancer. Her own old health problems had been in control; now, with his diagnosis, those problems seemed to increase, no longer in control but becoming more demanding. Her anxiety attacks returned; she couldn't sleep; her intestinal problems made her miserable. She tried bravely to keep her distress from her husband, but she discovered that, battling with her own pains and distress, she could not be there for him when he needed her most.

Just remember that the diagnosis of cancer shreds the illusion, for everyone, of being in control of one's own life and destiny. Uncertainty replaces a sense of order. Fear seeps in where only confidence existed before. Obviously and understandably, that happens to the person diagnosed with cancer, but fear and uncertainty have long arms. They inevitably embrace more than a single person, grabbing those—close family, lovers, extended family, friends, even coworkers—with any connection to the person involved.

Fear often shows up in odd, seemingly unrelated ways.

Lou Ellen's response to her sister-in-law's diagnosis of breast cancer was to experience a full-blown panic reaction. Lou Ellen became obsessed not about her breasts but about moles on her body, repeatedly questioning dermatologists about her risk of developing melanoma.

You will feel much more in control when you understand the powerful effects cancer has on your family and friends. This understanding allows you to help others through their pains and distress as well as to mobilize their energies on your own behalf. It is not easy to find the strength to reach out in your time of distress, but it is a generosity of spirit that multiplies manyfold as it returns to you.

All families will react to the illness, but not all families are alike. They can differ in many basic ways. You must look thoughtfully at what sort of family you belong to, what dynamics keep you together or push you apart. Families, like individuals, pass through different stages of development. A new family is not likely to handle a cancer crisis in the same way as a long-established family. In most instances familiarity breeds help and assistance. If you are part of a new family, you will understandably have to work doubly hard to establish or maintain truly open communication. If you are part of an old family, you may have to work even harder to break old, not always useful, patterns and relationships.

Cecilia was engaged to be married and only twenty-seven years old when her brain tumor was diagnosed. The wedding plans were deferred not only to accommodate her needs for surgery and chemotherapy, but for Cecilia and her fiancée to reevaluate their relationship and their commitment, and to deal with the complex reactions of their families

to her illness. Responding unusually well to treatments for her cancer and to the personal challenges they both faced, they set a new date for the wedding and married one year later.

Families differ in how strongly they are influenced by religious beliefs, the media, and others in the community. The degree of influence is often determined by which source provides the most believed information and the greatest comfort to family members. If you and others gather primary information from different sources, conflicts may be inevitable based on both literal differences in the information and the manner in which it is received. Do your best to anticipate them. For example, if you don't share the same religious or spiritual base, disharmony may follow. If one of you believes everything a particular information source reports and the other doesn't, friction between you, rather than enlightenment, may result. Acceptance of differences goes a long way toward preserving relationships.

Belinda was very devout in her religious beliefs. When her brother became ill with cancer, she became angry, confused, and more than a little depressed. She loved him so much. She also loved God. She believed in a personal God, an omnipotent God. How could her brother's illness be, as some said to her, the will of God? If these people were correct, how could she still love God? Happily, Belinda found an excellent pastoral counselor. The counseling process helped her resolve her confusion, lift her depression, and even some of her anger disappeared.

Some families are relatively closed off to non–family members and influences. They seem content to function without intimate involvement with outsiders. Consequently they appear less vulnerable to disruption by external events. Their relative self-sufficiency and clannishness may, however, make them more brittle and vulnerable when faced with an internal crisis. Their mutual dependence may be fine in normal times; it may be a problem in others.

Ellen adored her husband. His diagnosis of metastatic prostate cancer made her even more ferociously protective of him than ever. She fought the doctors constantly about informing him of the extent of his disease. She wanted only to protect him from the implications of the information, she said.

Still other families have permitted few barriers to grow between themselves and their community. They mingle easily and invite contact with others. These families often pride themselves on their flexibility and problem-solving abilities and, depending on the nature of the challenges presented, may have great capacities for adaptation to traumatic stress. They allow an easy flow of ideas, beliefs, and feelings into themselves and expression of their feelings outward. They are often open to wide ranges of information, consultation, and shared experience. These families may bond with nonrelated individuals, receiving support and assistance from them. If this appeals to you, but has not been part of your family style, realize that family patterns develop over many years, and don't look for that attitude to develop suddenly at your urging after a diagnosis.

Don, a brilliant journalist, was diagnosed with Hodgkin's lymphoma. He was only thirty-two years old. His bride of several months, his family and her family, and his supervisors at work all rallied to help him with his challenge. They reassured him of his position at work, assisted him in finding the best treatment program for his illness, and supported him in his decision to store his sperm before treatments began and in other decisions. They worked at being supportive but not interfering, assisting him only when assistance was called for or asked for. Within a year he was back at work with almost normal energy. His marriage had grown in mutual commitment, and he and his wife were discussing and planning for a pregnancy.

Families differ in how they listen or react to outside forces. How family members function with each other is not always the same within the family either. In some instances the shared burden may bring a family closer together, at least if you are among the lucky ones, but a cancer diagnosis can also make existing communication problems worse, leaving emotions raw and misunderstandings more likely. You may find yourself sharing information selectively, not completely, out of good intentions. You may keep information from others because you believe that you must protect or not bother them. Or you may pretend that discomforts do not exist out of fear of being seen as weak or needy. You may assume that others should know but not bother to inform them. It is hard work, but necessary work, to move yourself and your family toward directness and openness about information and feelings. You must have the courage to hear the feelings and opinions of others, even when they differ from your own.

Tony, age ten, knew it was a scary thing to have cancer. He had certainly suffered enough from the different medical tests and treatments as well as from having to drop out of sports and be absent from school so much. He also knew that his parents wanted him to believe he would be well soon. They were always saying things about how well he was doing and asking him how he was feeling. They just never asked him what he was feeling or what he knew about his illness. He actually had read his chart. He also heard the doctors talking on their rounds. He knew he might not live, but he loved his parents and wanted them to feel good. So he never told them what he knew. They pretended. He pretended. Pretending is hard work and uses energy better used in other ways.

Some family members, unable to deal with your illness, may withdraw. That isolation often leads to anger, a sense by you and others that the person doesn't care. That may not be the case at all. Caring and communicating that feeling at a particular moment may be beyond the emotional equipment of those involved.

What tormented Bob most was the deception, the lie. For some reason his whole family accepted the lie that he was not dying but was sim-

ply ill. If he would only keep quiet and undergo treatment, something good would result. He felt this falsity around him and within him. It did more to separate him from everyone and poison his last days than anything else.

Some families that do draw together may then isolate themselves from their community, from neighbors, from their church, from their normal activities. In the old days many people avoided talking of cancer as though there was something shameful about it. Indeed, fear generated stigma and kept it alive. Today, with awareness of cancer as widespread as it is, we are better at facing it, knowing that cancer is simply another difficult chronic illness no more shameful than a common cold. But some families still barricade themselves from the outside world, an action that does no one any good.

Even talking about "family" today requires some definition. Just a few decades ago a traditional family was made up of two parents, children, and other close relatives generally living close together, at least in the same town or community, if not on the same block. An extended family might include close friends who also offered emotional and, sometimes, material support. But families today are not what they once were. Today's world is a vastly different one.

Kids no longer go to college at the closest public university; they may marry someone they meet at a distant school and end up working and living far away. The need for work, regardless of schooling, may take us far from where we grew up. Families split, and children may end up living far from a sick parent and be estranged to some extent. Even loving, close-knit families may find members scattered from one corner of our country, or the world, to another. Our easy mobility, our spreading like leaves in the wind, imposes extraordinary emotional, economic, and logistical challenges to family as its members struggle to communicate and support one another while living hundreds, even thousands, of miles apart.

Close or far, self-contained or open, what is of primary importance is how family members communicate with one another, particularly now. So it is important to look at your family carefully, to take an inventory of relationships. It may be a struggle to define your family system and the relationships among its different members, but it is worth the struggle. It not only takes your mind off yourself for a moment but brings things into a clearer and more helpful focus.

Consider age differences. A family is likely to involve two or three generations. Where there are small children, there are problems of knowing what the child can usefully understand. To deny most children, of almost any age, any information is not helpful. They need to know that someone—mother, father, grandmother, grandfather, brother, sister—is ill. Or, if they are the patient, they need to know about their own illnesses.

Be alert to a child's needs. He or she may not yet understand death and may not even be interested in ultimate outcome so much as whether the affected person can play as before or read to the child, or take the child to the zoo.

Diana, age five, was at home one year after her diagnosis of leukemia, chatting with her mother. "Mommy," she said, "when you had leukemia as a little girl, did you get so many needles and bone marrows?"

Most younger children are basically concerned with their own little universe, of which we are only a part. Even when a child is the patient, his or her perspective arises from the world as understood by the child. So adjust the child's burdens to his or her age and understanding without hiding basic information and keep your expectations and responses in line with the age of the child.

Even preteen children may think of themselves first and how the illness affects their lives. "If Daddy dies, who will support us?" "Will I still be able to go to college?" "Are you dying, Mommy?" Everyone in a family must guard against taking offense at such naively direct and therefore, to the minds of adults, insensitive questions. Those personal concerns represent anxious, uncertain feelings. When those questions are dealt with, children will be concerned about the person with cancer and should not be shielded from the pain the entire family feels, which they really cannot escape. You can properly tell a child you don't know the answers to his or her questions when you in fact don't know. But to deceive children believing you are protecting them is to deceive yourself and to serve them poorly.

Adult children as well as nonadult children experience, in the context of your illness, a shifting of relationships. Needs for their time, support, and attention have changed. Appropriate responses require them to reevaluate their behavior toward you and their own expectations of themselves as well as of you. You find yourself faced with questions of what to tell them. You wonder about how you should tell them about your illness; you even wonder what they need to know. You struggle with thoughts about protecting them from worries and additional burdens, while you simultaneously may find yourself wishing that they would help more without having to be asked.

The reverse side of the age coin is the effort to protect even older generations. "Don't tell Grandpa. It would kill him." "If Mama found out, she'd just die." Most adults, in full command of their senses, will soon figure out that something is wrong and will resent the fact that they were not told when others were. Most adults have survived other shocks in their lives. Honesty here is just as vital as it is with children.

How you share your frightening or troublesome condition is vital, too. When information is shared, that sharing should be straightforward, direct, and as unburdened by emotional displays as possible. Even in families where that has not always been the habit or style, it is important to reach for that tone. The alternative invites focusing on and remembering the emotions rather than the information. This sets up both you and your family members for future misunderstandings.

There is something more to consider. Your position and role in your family influence the responses of the whole family as a unit as well as the individuals within it. Whatever your position, you should recall your relationship with the family and its various members before you became ill and note how it has changed.

Are you a breadwinner, a spouse, primary homemaker, or dependent?

Dan and Pat had been married for thirty-five years when his cancer was diagnosed. Their marriage worked quite well during those years. She ran the home and took primary responsibility for raising the children while he invested himself in his career and the income it provided for the family. Now he was home, and she was helping make ends meet through a full-time job in the community. Both found themselves, in a reversal of roles, increasingly irritable and discouraged by the changes.

Some Specific Effects of Cancer on Families

Your particular family may not have serious preexisting problems that make it more difficult to cope. But many families do. The problems may be economic; they may involve generally strained marital relations, specific marital problems, or divorce; they may involve other chronic illnesses or disabilities; or they may involve substance abuse, abusive behavior, or serious mental illness. Families with problems often experience a cancer diagnosis as the straw that breaks the camel's back. An explosion of emotions may occur—instead of gathering resources and mobilizing support, the experience becomes an additional destructive force in family relationships.

The atmosphere in a family functioning poorly is not conducive to healing. When normal functioning is disrupted by illness, there is a dramatic absence of support or, worse, the acting out of clearly unhelpful behavior (economic irresponsibility, infidelity, psychological abuse). Family members become alienated from one another, and the family is forever changed by the encounter with cancer.

Patty, a married architect with two children, was receiving the best in medical care. Patty's parents never showed their feelings. They were masters of polite conversation, of doing the socially correct thing, but their emotions were always masked in a frozen smile. So when she developed bowel cancer at a relatively young age, they went into a frenzy of activity, but they did everything with exclusive reference to themselves. Patty kept her parents informed, but they did not know how to respond, how to share, how to talk. So their visits were always painful and exhausting. They would never ask how she was or talk, in any other way, about her cancer. They would just create lists and bustle about her house fixing and painting things they hadn't been asked to fix or paint, vacuuming, and rearranging furniture. In their inarticulate panic they created discomfort for everyone.

Caroline couldn't wait for her husband's retirement. It was then that she planned to tell him and the children that she was leaving. Caroline wanted so badly to spend her late middle age and older years out of her marriage and away from what had become the awfulness of him. She focused so much on these plans that she skipped her physical examination for two years. By the time her lack of energy drove her to the doctor, her cancer had spread. Her diagnosis was like a cruel joke, dashing all hope for her dreams.

What you hope for is that no matter what your family dynamics, no matter what your own role, your family will find the strength to cope. That means finding ways to support one another emotionally for sure, financially when necessary and possible, dealing honestly with one another during a difficult time. As the disease progresses to remission or stabilization, the crisis for the family should resolve itself. Members can then shift their attention back to ongoing interests, involvements, and activities. Well-functioning families allow this shift to occur while they remain quite capable of remobilizing their resources for any new crisis that may occur.

Yet the absence of emotional upsets and misunderstandings is not by itself the same as excellent coping. To cope with adversity at the highest levels, you must accept that some kinds of unhappiness may occur. After all, life's normal problems—not life threatening, but often serious nonetheless—do not disappear in times of prolonged crisis or challenge. Cancer and its treatments simply create special and additional challenges. They must all be dealt with.

What coping at the highest level means is that despite normal ups and downs in functioning and happiness, the sense of support expressed in both attitude and action continues to be there when you need it. That support can include many ordinary things: driving you to appointments, being available to listen without imposing advice or judgments on what you should be doing that you are not, shopping for you, helping with meal preparations, helping with child care, helping with organizing and paying bills; and providing housekeeping assistance. Support may also include major assistance such as donations of blood, blood platelets, or even bone marrow.

In response to the demands of treatments, the communication, responsibilities, and uses of personal energy within families all change. This change is influenced significantly by the extent to which you find yourself and your family emotionally dependent on the medical system during treatment. In addition to the medical system, other parts of the human service system (including social services and psycho-oncology services) may be grafted into your family. They have to be reckoned with as they affect relationships within the family.

Families quickly learn much of the jargon of the medical system. Family members most involved in helping join you by learning their way around the medical system and learning how to make it more responsive to your care and other needs.

Bob's treatment was complete. It had been a rocky road with several different treatments and complications of infections before he finally went

into complete remission. He had spent an extensive amount of time at the medical center both as an inpatient and in the clinics. Finally, discharged to long-term follow-up, Bob found himself strangely anxious. Was he safe without being seen every week? How did he know that his body was all right without the frequent blood tests? He missed the comforting voices of certain doctors and nurses. To his astonishment, he discovered that even the smells of the medical center and the appearance of the buildings had become important parts of his life. Without all of that he was not sure he was quite right. He found himself making up reasons to drive by the medical center every week because it somehow made him feel better.

Your closest family members join you in developing skills to assure that doctors and nurses and their associates perform better for you and that errors are not made. These skills include showing personal interest in the individual health professionals; this helps enhance their personal interest in you. Skills applied may include the development of capacities to regularly stroke the egos of medical professionals through compliments about their dedication, cleverness, responsiveness, and caring.

Emotionally healthy family members give themselves the freedom, in private as well as with you directly, to express their reactions to your diagnosis. Whether they are your own children (all ages) or parents or spouses, or siblings or cousins, they have their own anger and depressive reactions. There are many emotional struggles and conditions to deal with: not thinking clearly, anxiety and tension, guilt, fear, sleep problems. Maintaining hope for you is tough for them, and, on the other hand, it is easy for family members to feel isolated from acquaintances and friends who seem to have no serious problems, certainly none that are life threatening.

It is even possible that family members, without realizing it, will feel hostility toward you because they will be receiving less attention than you. Sometimes family members act out these feelings, most commonly through silent unexplained withdrawal or by bombarding you with unsolicited advice about new treatments or making excessive, repetitive inquiries about your health.

If you have siblings, no matter their age or yours, their emotional responses to your diagnosis will be intense. Siblings worry about you; they also worry about themselves. They ask themselves, "Why not me? When will it be me? Is it contagious or genetic? Will I get it, too?" The answer is never clear or satisfying, and your siblings will find themselves musing about death. Their age does, of course, color both the extent and exact nature of these musings. Depending on the personalities of your siblings and your relationship with one another, they may or may not reveal any of these thoughts to you. But understand that they are there and that they are not selfish, mean-spirited, or belittling of you. How they behave is just part, however aggravating at times, of the normal range of responses to cancer in a family.

There is another fact that is inescapable. It is normal for siblings to have had periods of difficulty and anger with one another. We all do, and those feelings stir up, if only for a moment, thoughts or hopes that another person would disappear, run away, or even die. Those feelings may have occurred yesterday or years and years ago. They may have been forgotten until this crisis when they well up anew, influencing behaviors in ways such as a slowness to respond to your requests for help, irritable outbursts toward you, and even avoidance of you. So remember that your siblings are who they are as the result of their accumulated feelings and personality. Don't expect them to respond in ways significantly different from what you know them to be—if they were open and caring before, they will likely be that way now; if they were distant and incapable of generous love before, they are not likely to change much now.

Yet, having said that, you can expect that your illness will bring out a variety of reactions, some that you expect and some that you don't. Your siblings will respond to both your visible reactions and your nonverbal signals. They will see your expressions of pain. They will notice your weakness, fatigue, or nausea. They will notice changes in appetite and weight. They will see the side effects of treatment as well as the impact of the disease.

Ryan sends this brief e-mail message about his chemotherapy treatments: "Well, friends, I am living much the same life I have always lived, counting the dreams that flee from my grasp, and when I run out of these I can count the hairs that are falling from my head."

At least initially as they see you become diminished from your preillness state, they will respond with sadness, fear, and the frustration of being limited in what they can do. They may set about seeking explanations from medicine and religion for what has happened to you. Sometimes the fruits of their searches are shared and truly of help to you; sometimes their searches are a purely private excursion for themselves but one that provides them the strength to continue at your side. Sometimes when they do share, you may not like what they have to report.

If you approach sibling relationships from the point of view that you are ill and they ought to be there for you fully, unquestioningly, and as you need them, without regard to your past relationships and their personalities, you are bound to be disappointed. Even at this moment those relationships must be based on understanding, reality, and mutual concern. To be understood requires that you be understanding as well. Sometimes, faced with the crisis of cancer, siblings who have old, unresolved resentments do talk them through, attaining new levels of communication as well as of understanding. You should allow for hopefulness about relationships simultaneously with your hopefulness about dealing with your cancer.

If you have a spouse, he or she will be touched by your illness in ways similar to those of siblings, but even more so. How you get along now will be influenced by the kind of relationship you had before becoming ill, how close your friendship was, how great your trust, how intense and accepted your interdependence, the ages of your children, the relationship you have with them. The rhythms and priorities of your spouse's life are changed as he or she focuses on assisting you and at least initially taking on increased responsibilities in the maintenance of all aspects of your home, family, and personal finance. It becomes a time when marriage vows and personal values are truly tested, when the patient and spouse reap the rewards or pain of their prior accumulated years of collaboration, communication, and expressions of love.

To Cindy, her husband, Art, was a heroic figure. He had immense energy and intellect. Successful in business and athletics, he gave large amounts of time to the community. But he avoided doctors and ignored symptoms. When his widespread cancer was diagnosed, her anger at him for his self-neglect was immense. Wisely, she sought help for these disturbing feelings through psychotherapy. This freed her to use her energy during their remaining time together to talk, to parent together, to weep together, to fight the ravages of illness.

So, whatever your family condition—new or old, cheerful and friendly or difficult and argumentative, economically well off or in tight financial circumstances, close at hand or widely scattered, closely knit or barely family, there are things for you to do. Let's look at some of them, many implicit in what we have been talking about, but well worth repeating.

Action Steps for Family Survival

The most powerful way to achieve the surrounding family atmosphere you need, after you have gotten your second opinions and agreed to a particular recommended course of treatment, is to convene in your home or apartment a meeting of your closest family members and most intimate friends. On your own turf, inform them of your illness as you understand it. This minimizes the distortions of second- and thirdhand information that are bound to occur. (Remember the telephone game of childhood where a simple whispered sentence turns into something quite different from how it began?) Medical information, particularly in times of crisis, has an even stronger tendency to change from fact to fantasy.

Your meeting becomes your own news conference, where you can explain about the treatments you are having or are about to start. Then explain the different ways you believe they can be helpful to you. Don't order them. Don't command. Simply list, as conversationally as you can, examples: driving you on certain days to the clinic or hospital, picking up children, walking the dog, preparing a meal, explaining your situation and needs to others. Before asking for questions, give those gathered with you some guidance about how you want them to check up on you, how you want them to inquire about your well-being.

Not giving family and friends guidance in this area results in one of the greatest stresses for cancer patients—the constant but unpredictable well-meaning questions about how you are and how you are doing. Unbridled, these inquiries, frequently made in awkward, uncomfortable ways, become disruptive, irritating intrusions into private moments, draining your patience and energies.

You want people to be interested, helpful, and supportive. Family members and friends just need to be taught *how* to do this for *you*. Sometimes self-satire helps.

Paul writes a letter, which he photocopies and mails out. The letter starts: "Dear Friends and Relations: Unfortunately, the drugs that produce the cure also produce side effects that could be classified under the general heading of Instant Aging. I have developed incipient baldness, dry skin rashes, irregularity, and the posture and gait of a retired British admiral with an old wound. It certainly has been an instructive experience to face death eyeball to eyeball (when death could get his eyeball under the pillow, which I kept firmly pressed over my head the whole time in the hospital)."

What feels comfortable and right is different for each of us. This is one area in which you, as a cancer patient, can truly empower yourself and take control while simultaneously being very helpful to others, for no one is quite sure what to do, what is right until given such guidance.

But even before you gather your family, there are basic things for you to do. Identify vulnerable areas that exist for you and your family. To do so you need to examine the following:

- Look at the communication styles of family members, considering siblings, children, parents, grandparents, and other more distant but perhaps very involved relatives.
- Review stressful life events of the past and how you have coped with them not only personally but within your family.
- Identify current stresses on the family—from community commitments to economic problems to other health problems that may exist in addition to the cancer diagnosis.
- Pay attention to how the diagnosis and treatments have currently knocked the family system or other members off track with respect to work, education, community involvement, and responsibilities. Even little changes involving things such as tasks family members are no longer making time for as they assist you can accumulate to the point of becoming important stressors.

You need to identify, even list on a piece of paper for yourself and for the family, current stresses that may relate to past experiences. These include economic problems or outright poverty; other health problems that you or your close family members have suffered, especially any experiences with severe chronic illnesses and most especially experiences with cancer in a sibling, parent, or child;

alcohol or substance abuse problems; chronic marital discord; chronic problems with minor or adult children; psychological problems that noticeably impaired your quality of life and functioning; migrant lifestyle (including that led by employees of large corporations and government agencies). Identifying the important stresses in your life becomes your first step toward improved coping and regaining an improved sense of control. You don't want to fight old battles or settle scores, but it is important to understand all of the emotional baggage you and your family carry and must deal with. Think through what you are dealing with. A little history lesson can be a good thing.

Stressful life events from the past may have produced vulnerabilities for the present. Perhaps they had been mastered by the family, giving it a sense that it can surmount almost any problem with the right kind of effort and help. Frequently the mastery of past major stressful events involves putting unhappy or upsetting things out of mind. This psychological coping technique is probably used to some degree by everyone and in all families. Unfortunately it produces vulnerabilities in the present, when we encounter situations that remind us of times when we felt frightened, out of control, lost, helpless, even hopeless, or somehow responsible for some unhappy event.

An example involves the family that suffered the loss of a child from some form of cancer. Fears that the child's cancer is somehow connected to angry feelings or other imagined or real transgressions were suppressed long ago. But these uneasy feelings may suddenly come rushing back into the awareness of the family at the time you are diagnosed as having cancer. For those families in which this happens, feelings are often associated with uncomfortable thoughts that the current illness is punishment for forgotten events of the past.

Finally, in good days and bad, your family is a vital bridge to people and institutions—churches, synagogues, mosques, fraternal or cultural groups—in your community. In addition, professional and support groups are there to be of help when asked. Your family can be the way to connect with all the energy that can be turned to making your quality of life so much better. Any of the problems I have posed in this chapter that are unresolved, causing grief you don't need, can probably be diminished, if not eliminated, by a resource nearby.

Begin with the American Cancer Society, a Visiting Nurses Association, and marriage and family counseling centers, which may provide information, counseling, transportation, companions, or equipment.

There are cancer advocacy groups—Coalition of Cancer Survivors, The Candlelighters, CanSurmount, and Y-ME among others—that are set up to provide or direct you to support for families in various forms of distress.

If you have belonged to groups like the American Legion, the Veterans of Foreign Wars, or the Eagles or Elks, you know they often have volunteers who are there to help families in distress. You may even have been a volunteer yourself. And virtually every community has clinical social workers, clergy trained in counseling, clinical nurse practitioners, psychologists, and psychiatrists who can be there when you need them.

Let me end with only this suggestion. When you seek help from organizations or individual practitioners for family problems, maintain reasonable vigilance combined with common sense. You don't always get what you want or need, so be a careful consumer of helping services. Preserving your autonomy and integrity must be your guiding passion.

You should not think of your family as seeking help to be fixed in some general way. You should be resolving some specific, defined problem. Never allow the family to feel itself the helpless victim, the supplicant totally dependent on the generosity of others. That route leads to surrender and a kind of psychosocial, even spiritual, death. Whatever problems your family is faced with must be visualized as problems; problems are challenges; problems can either be lessened or solved. You seek help and assistance in that process.

But you must see yourself and help your family to see itself as having a significant role in meeting the challenges. In that way you get better specific results, and you all handle the crisis of cancer more positively.

Finally, if you find that there are family members, friends, or acquaintances who are not dealing with you respectfully and intelligently; if the support and treatments, wherever they come from, do not make sense to you or, after a reasonable time, are not accomplishing the goals you want, you must assert yourself. You must set limits. If you feel irritation, disappointment, even anger, don't disguise it. Evaluate it, reflect on it, then act on it, directing that action toward improving your quality of life. Help, even the best intentioned, when it is intrusive to the point of trying your patience, drains your energies, challenges your autonomy, and must be dealt with. If you do not, you will have the sense, once again, of losing control. The experience of losing control pushes your whole self into a hyperalert state—some form of fight-or-flight reaction. This works against the healing forces of your body, dampening the activity of your body's immune system. It also, by dissipating your energies in unneeded ways, diminishes your quality of life.

7 Community and Work

WE'VE TALKED in earlier chapters about how you should react after a diagnosis of cancer. We agreed, I hope, that you need to take control, to be in charge of yourself, your treatment, and your surroundings. We've talked about your family and how they can be a drain on your emotions or an immense help as you work your way on your passage, with good fortune, to remission or cure from the diagnosis of cancer. It is a difficult journey from confirmation of the diagnosis through treatment decisions and their implementation and side effects. That is a lot on your plate.

But there are several more things you must consider as you try to protect yourself in a difficult time. You need to think about what may happen at work and within your community. You may ask, "What can I do about what goes on at work? It's up to the boss. What can I do about my community? It's just there, and I am here, diagnosed with cancer." In fact you can influence both your workplace and your community. You can make them work for you. At least you can make sure they don't drain your energy and your spirit. You need to maintain the quality of your life as well as you can, and that means knowing what you will face.

Start with this. Anticipation and knowledge are valuable tools. Knowing what may occur means you can, at least in some important ways, handle the aggravations that almost inevitably come your way. Fear, rejection, and prejudice are the three "furies" of cancer you can expect to find in your community and at your workplace. You must be ready to handle each one of them. To be aware is to take the first step toward balancing the new burdens. Simply put, to be in control, there is information you should have and there are concerns to ponder about your workplace and fellow workers.

In the community, and the workplace as part of the community, there is frequently a mistaken assumption that the diagnosis of cancer is a death sentence and that the person who has cancer is somehow now unclean or unsafe to be with. That outrageous view continues to distort the truth and, in many cases, poison the immediate environment that surrounds you.

All this arises from the widespread lack of understanding about what cancers are and how and why they develop. It is fed by some things that are real—some, although certainly not all, cancer patients have lost strength and easy movement, changed posture, lost body hair from treatments. These visual signals encourage the fear of contagion that lives too frequently in people of ordinary goodwill. It often overshadows normal feelings of caring and compassion. Some people, for example, still believe that cancer evolves as punishment for past moral transgressions. (What an ugly distortion of the religious spirit that is!) You must have noticed some of these attitudes.

Most of us are not rich enough to avoid work. At least some of the time you may have to work even in illness, and you should want to. Keeping busy can be good medicine if done sensibly. But, as I have noted, the workplace of the day before your diagnosis and that of the day after are not the same.

You may experience everything from shunning to intolerance of absences for treatments to the reduction or removal of responsibilities because of the assumption you will be diminished not only during the illness and its treatments but permanently. Your situation is unique. How you handle your condition is special. But there is still a lot of ignorance out there about cancer and cancer patients that permits other people to impose on you expectations based on their ignorance.

Nina successfully attained a middle management position by the time she was thirty. Her salary was finally based on a yearly professional wage scale rather than hourly pay. Her work skills and ability to get along with her coworkers combined to make her a rising star in her boss's eyes. Then her house of cards tumbled rapidly: a lump in her cystic breasts proved cancerous. There was an inevitable burden on her energy and time as she sought a second opinion, decided on a treatment plan, and began treatment. She asked her boss to permit a more flexible scheduling of her work. His response was immediate and harsh: she was an abuser of privileges of her status and, therefore, unprofessional.

She was told that she must maintain her productivity in a "normal" fashion. When she failed to make her first postdiagnosis work deadline, her manager made snide comments about her work to other employees. Then, without discussion with her, work was withheld. In defense of herself she referred to written company policies. She was then accused of insubordination as well as abuse of goodwill. Fear of loss of income and benefits, extraordinary anxiety at the workplace, where she previously had felt so competent and assured, were now added to the anxiety, fear, and general stresses of cancer treatment.

Most of us define ourselves, at least partially, and are defined by the work we do, including children, whose work is in school. Ideally your work serves not merely as a source of income and benefits but as one of the reference points, one of the stabilizing and organizing forces in your life. Ideally, although this is not always the case, work serves in times of crisis as a significant source of comfort and support.

Nina's story is played out every day over and over again for both men and women; only the details are different. Supervisors are uninformed or indifferent to personnel policies or may even be encouraged by their own bosses to be "unaware" of the rules. It is not unheard of for inappropriate demands to be made on the employee and coworker hostility to be encouraged; then, using the turmoil as an excuse, demotions, denial of promotions, undesirable transfers, attempts to withhold pay, alteration of benefits, and even dismissal occur.

These actions exist not only in the pursuit of maintaining productivity and profitability at whatever cost but also in the context of widely held myths about those who have cancer. In 1991 a study found almost 50 percent of supervisors said that knowing that a job candidate had cancer would affect their decision to hire that person; 66 percent said that if an employee developed cancer, they would be actively concerned about whether or not the employee could still adequately perform his or her job. Thirteen percent of employees felt that a peer with cancer probably could not do the job; 25 percent anticipated having to work harder to pick up the slack for their fellow employee with cancer. Certainly many wonderful cases of caring and loving support exist in the workplace, but these figures reflect a combination of realistic concerns as well as erroneous attitudes that influence the behavior of supervisors and peers.

Faced with all this, you should be aware of protections afforded in the workplace by employer policies and county, state, and federal laws. These laws vary considerably, as do employer policies, so you must check carefully to determine your rights. Prospective employers may ask about your health (e.g., "Do you have a health problem or disability?") *only* if you have a *visible* disability that appears to the employer as one that might affect your job performance. The employer, however, may legally ask details about your disability only *after* you have been offered the job.

General protections requiring reasonable accommodation at the workplace and regulations against discrimination are guaranteed by federal law under the Federal Rehabilitation Act of 1973 and the Americans with Disabilities Act of 1992. These protections are directed at employers, employment agencies, and labor unions. However, they currently do not apply to organizations with fewer than fifteen employees, nor do they apply to uniformed members of the armed forces.

Reasonable accommodation to the demands of your illness and disability as required by law does *not* mean receiving paid leave beyond that granted by company policy. It also does not mean a total dropping of job-related performance expectations. Reasonable accommodation *does* mean negotiated flexible work hours, working from home when possible and appropriate, use of earned sick and vacation leave with pay, and use of unpaid leave. Under the Federal Family and Medical Leave Act (it applies currently only to employers of fifty or more people), after you have worked a minimum of twenty-five hours per week for one year, you are to be allowed job protection and benefits while on unpaid leave for up to twelve weeks for documented serious illness in yourself or a close family member. Corporations are allowed, however, to write policies that exempt the highest-paid employees from this protection.

If you are having a less-than-positive experience in the workplace, fight back. It may not win you friends at first, but you will gain self-respect and probably much more. Start by gathering information. Review your employer's written personnel and benefit policies. Obtain state and county regulations concerning illness, disabilities, and benefits. You may have grounds for a grievance within the company or beyond, such as with your state's Equal Employment Opportunity Commission (EEOC).

Some of you may encounter difficult situations in which you must confront your employer or seek assistance through the EEOC. Some of you may even encounter situations where legal guidance and even more aggressive legal action are required. Remember that if this comes to pass you should seek a quality lawyer through your local bar association, checking reputation and credentials with your union if you belong to one, and the local American Cancer Society. National advocacy organizations such as the National Coalition for Cancer Survivorship often can provide helpful insights and guidance through booklets developed by their volunteers and consultants. Selected references to these are found in Appendix E.

Many people with cancer today, or who have minor children with cancer, are well treated in their workplace. This, with any luck, is your reality. Even if it is, however, do not depend on others for all knowledge and guidance. Learn, as I have said, the basic employment and benefit policies of your company. If you belong to a union, read the contract policies concerning illness and disability. Get or have someone get the relevant local and state regulations covering your situation. Be realistic with yourself in consultation with your doctors and nurses about your energy levels and other realities that influence your ability to be at and to perform at work.

Then, with the assistance of others, try to be a force for cancer education with peers and supervisors at work, using your own experience as an example if you are comfortable doing so. While working, use flextime as creatively as possible to maintain high standards of both self-care and work performance.

The Smiths were delighted with the new home they had just located in a community outside the city. The streets were safe, the school district had a good reputation, and the houses were affordable. Their bid was accepted on the house. Then the troubles began. The agent called, informing them that the sellers and the bank(!) wondered if they would withdraw, even offering them a financial incentive to do so. Shocked, the Smiths inquired and discovered that influential members of the neighborhood association had learned that their ten-year-old son was a leukemia patient. They preferred not to have a child with leukemia in their neighborhood.

As difficult as your workplace can be, you may find your neighborhood and your daily and routine social relations more troublesome. Twenty-five years ago I worked with several families who were shocked to find potential neighbors organizing to prevent them from moving into a new neighborhood after learning that there was a child with leukemia. The fact that it was not contagious or in any other way disruptive to their own lives made no difference.

But your own friends and longtime neighbors may fail you as well. You may find that you are suddenly uninvited to social events and no longer invited to homes of previously friendly people. The neighborhood barbecue goes on without you; the swimming party is canceled; the soccer car pool is suddenly too full to accommodate you. These rejections are hard to take but harder to prevent or avoid. Think ahead about what you will do if they do happen. Doing something, at least speaking up, is often better than suffering indignities in silence.

At first friends and neighbors of Bob and Jan demonstrated great interest when Bob was diagnosed with colon cancer. But as he progressed through his treatments—surgery with placement of a colostomy; chemotherapies that took away his vigor, changed his skin color, decreased the energy with which he walked and talked—the telephone calls and spontaneous visits offering assistance, providing an occasional food dish, inquiring about his health all slowed down considerably. Jan then began to notice as the months went by that the usual invitations to social events as well as spontaneous invitations to the homes of friends and neighbors evaporated.

While such rejection still occurs often throughout the United States, some positive changes are taking place. Through the efforts of the late philanthropist Mary Lasker, the American Cancer Society, and the many other cancer advocacy groups that evolved after World War II, change in attitude about cancer was encouraged, and much of it has taken root, although slowly. People talk more openly about their cancers these days than ten years ago. Public figures in a variety of fields have come forward to acknowledge their cancers: that they have fought cancer and remain active and successful. Mrs. Nelson "Happy" Rockefeller was an early celebrity who spoke out. That tradition of honesty and openness has been continued by Betty Ford, Norman Schwarzkopf, Bob Dole, Hubert H. Humphrey, and Gilda Radner, among others.

This increasing openness brings with it, in many cases, a lessening of stigma and rejection. It allows your community to become what it should be for you and your family: more of a resource, more of a source of support. Today you are far from alone. In the United States alone there are more than ten million individuals with cancer. You and your immediate family are a clearly noticeable new minority in our culture. More than four million cancer patients have been living with their diagnosis and its attendant uncertainty for more than five years.

Be active with respect to your community. In this way you will contribute to your quality of life, that of your family, and that of other cancer patients. You can muster some energy during treatment, and definitely afterward, to join efforts in educating others about your illness, including how to be of help and how not to be of help. Those you come in contact with can learn from your example that cancer is a chronic illness, not an inevitable and immediate passport to withdrawal and death. Any anxiety others may feel about relating to someone with an illness or about possible contagion can be channeled into activities that support both you and the efforts to educate others to treat cancer as any other disease.

The resources available to you and your family are extensive. Find a nearby local branch of the American Cancer Society. Learn if your community has an advocacy organization for your particular kind of cancer and, if not, whether there is a national organization. Contact or have a family member contact the National Coalition for Cancer Survivorship as well as the information service of the National Cancer Institute for their lists of publications and notable events.

If you are part of a religious congregation or community service organization, enlist the group in helping with education about cancer directed toward your immediate community. Often knowledgeable speakers can be obtained from local hospitals or medical societies.

For those who are computer literate and have access to the Internet, vast amounts of information about all aspects of cancer are available. A caution here, though. There is no quality control on much, if not most, of the information. Seeing it on the screen in front of you doesn't make it necessarily true or helpful. Indeed, if you don't consider what you read with care, it can be harmful. Computer chat lines also exist, presenting a new form of community and support. In Appendix E you will find listings of some of the best electronic resources available.

There are, in short, many places and institutions of assistance within your community. Making sure you make use of some of the resources that are there adds importantly to your survivorship. Local and national cancer advocacy organizations, religious congregations, community service organizations, antidiscrimination laws, and disability protection laws make up some of the many protective resources within our communities. A supportive community helps buffer you from the tendency of all of us when under long-term, severe stress to negatively interpret personal experiences and the behavior of others. A supportive community helps you cope with the severe economic impact of nonreimbursable home care costs, health aides, transportation costs, unreimbursed medical costs, lost income, and lost income opportunities. A supportive community helps reduce your isolation from others and actively increase social contact. In summary, a supportive community helps maintain quality of life and realistic hope.

The importance of community is articulated for all of us in Natalie Davis Spingarn's Cancer Survivors Bill of Rights, endorsed by the American Cancer Society. All of us should be aware of its four main points:

1. Survivors have the right to assurance of lifelong medical care as needed.
2. In their personal lives, survivors, like other Americans, have the right to the pursuit of happiness.
3. In the workplace survivors have the right to equal job opportunities.
4. Since health insurance is an overriding survivorship concern, every effort should be made to assure all survivors adequate health insurance, whether public or private.

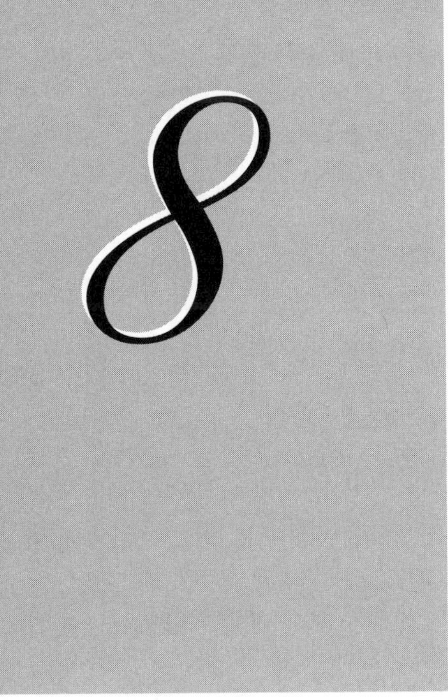

The Costs of Treatment and Insurance

THIS IS AN UGLY CHAPTER, and I wish I didn't have to write it. It's about money. In fact it is somewhat easier to talk about cancer and its health consequences than it is to talk about economic consequences. Health care insurance in the United States is a mess. For most cancer patients (and families) the expense is substantial, and health insurance does not always cover all of it. Personal savings may be eaten up. Sick leave is swallowed like a gulp of air. One burden is piled on another in what seems like a never-ending trial. It is the last thing you want to think about after a diagnosis, but you have to if you are to survive, not physically but economically.

If the patient is a child, costs involve lost work time by parents and increased demands for help that must be paid for. This help may involve paying for assistance in child care, housekeeping, shopping, or transportation. These costs too often can add up to as much as one-third of an average family's income!

If the patient is a parent, the other parent—if there are two—must to some extent take up the responsibilities of the parent receiving treatment and work harder, dealing with any increased family expenses as well as any lost income that may result.

If you are the patient, you may not have large amounts of accumulated sick leave available. You may not have short-term disability insurance. Thus cancer may demand traumatic changes in the use and flow of economic resources. For many, perhaps for you too, cancer literally requires various forms of personal belt tightening.

Tammy and John felt fortunate to have health insurance that covered, after a $500 deductible, 100 percent of the hospital costs for treatment of their teenage son Billy's sarcoma. Ten months into his treatment course they were astounded to find themselves looking at a second mortgage on their home or loans against John's retirement account. Time in and out of hospital spent with or on behalf of Billy, keeping up with the needs of their two younger children, forced both Tammy and John to take some leave without pay from their jobs. They also needed to hire part-time help with the home. They needed to pay out of pocket for some of Billy's postsurgical rehabilitation needs. Lost income and unpredicted costs had accumulated to thousands of dollars!

What could Jose do? At twenty-four years old he was a pretty good carpenter. He never had trouble finding a job as a freelancer. He believed that when he got older he would need health insurance but that for the moment coverage for accidents by those who hired him was sufficient. However, a sore throat and swollen neck that wouldn't go away led him to see his parents' doctor. He told Jose that he had Hodgkin's disease, a form of cancer. It could be cured if Jose acted fast. Jose was in a panic: how would he pay for even the further diagnostic tests needed, much less the treatment?

Max, at sixty-seven years old, responded well to the chemotherapy for his bowel cancer. He was grateful for his apparent improvement using his oncologist's three-drug regimen. Then an upsetting event happened: a letter from his insurance company informed him that one of the drugs prescribed by his doctor was "off-label," meaning that the Physicians' Desk Reference *did not list this medicine for primary use in Max's disease. Therefore, the insurance company wrote, it would not pay for this medicine; it would pay for the other two. For Max this meant an additional $50 per week of out-of-pocket expenses—a financial stretch for him. He wondered if the insurance company knew something about the treatment of his condition that his doctor did not know. For the first time his confidence in his doctor was shaken. Should he continue to trust his doctor's judgment? If he did, how could he explain to the doctor, his family, and his friends the financial distress this would cause? Would he still be able to make ends meet?*

The Impact of Costs

A 1994 study found an extraordinary economic impact on patients with severe illness, including cancers, and their families. Despite the fact that 96 percent of those studied had health insurance, 31 percent lost most of their life savings. The money went to pay for nonreimbursable costs such as home care, home health aides, transportation, and medicines not covered by insurance. In addition, 29 percent of the families lost income and as a result had to make personal life changes ranging from finding a smaller home to delaying education or other personal care needs. The population of patients was not an old one—55 percent were under age sixty-five. Indeed, the younger the patient with a major illness, the greater the economic burden on the family.

Our Distorted Values

Health care in our free-market setting is considered a commodity rather than a basic responsibility of society. Commodities are bought and sold for profit, in health care increasingly and devastatingly so. A wise professor, Robert T. Rubin, described the situation precisely: "The bottom line of the balance sheet is the supreme datum."

Unlike most other industrialized nations, we do not guarantee health care to our citizens. Unfortunately only in the United States do private companies run the health insurance system, handle your claims, and decide what is covered and what is not. Virtually everyone agrees that we have a problem of immense proportion. Recent efforts to resolve this problem sensibly and equitably and to control extraordinary escalation in health care costs have yielded some positive changes. We have also, however, stepped back toward the abyss of cancer and other chronic diseases equaling personal bankruptcy and toward more and more restrictions on care. What all this means is that you must deal with a maze when you should be maintaining your energy, strength, and focus on getting well.

It is a troublesome prospect. In short, health care costs and how they are met through the various forms of health care programs (health insurance, health maintenance organizations, other health plans, Medicare, Medicaid, CHAMPUS/Tricare) becomes another challenge as well as another potential threat to the quality of life and well-being of any cancer patient. In looking at the often-praised health maintenance organizations, a special 1996 *Consumer Reports* study found that 18 percent of HMO members pursued medical care outside to obtain treatment they felt was necessary but unavailable within the HMO.

Bills for diagnostic tests, surgery, radiation treatments, chemotherapy, supportive and rehabilitative surgeries can all become mountainous sources of stress and distress. Particularly when hospitalizations are involved, bills can pursue families for months or years afterward, peppering the family with demands for payment and threats of bad credit ratings. And sometimes they come from errors in billing as well as from services really rendered.

Errors in Billing

Errors sometimes include billings for procedures, even surgeries, not performed. Errors include bills for the mistakes of technicians or inadequate doctor-technician communication. A good example is being sent for an MRI with contrast and having the MRI done but no contrast substance given. When that is discovered, the patient is sent back for a second MRI, this time actually receiving the contrast material, and then is billed for both procedures.

You need to understand and check the accuracy of hospital bills and then check them again. Understand the explanation of benefits forms (EOBs) sent by insurance companies or their representatives. They don't make it easy for you. Work with these EOBs as guides to payment of services, understanding what is and what is not covered by insurance. Even with understanding you may find that all this extra work becomes a major source of psychological distress, frequently requiring months to straighten out what should be a simple problem. You are not being paranoid if you sometimes feel the insurance company is determined to outlast your attention and energy.

You are discovering that coverage for all medical costs is far from universal. And even if you do have coverage through an insurance company, managed care company, or HMO, you may encounter difficulty if the diagnostic procedures needed or the treatments sought are beyond the standard normal treatments approved by that particular insurer. (That approval may not relate to the highest-quality treatment recommended by experts in your form of cancer!) Legal disputes are increasing with the various managed care companies that design their reimbursements to maximize their profits around the least expensive common accepted treatments. These companies refuse, except under duress (that is, when threatened with legal action or actually challenged in court) to pay for cutting-edge or unusual but traditional medical treatments even for major problems.

They also frequently and successfully refuse to pay for requested nontraditional forms of treatment or cutting-edge diagnostic evaluations such as genetic screening.

Many of these companies try in various ways to inhibit your physicians from informing you about treatment alternatives because of their greater cost. They also, as mentioned earlier, are more and more often refusing to pay for off-label uses of medicines despite the reality in clinical practice that such use has been a successful and innovative part of the art of medicine for decades.

We Need a Consumer Revolution Now!

Actually, your situation may be much worse than I've described. We really need a call to arms, a call for a consumer-led revolution against the current, expanding free-market forces that by now have taken over at least 60 percent of the health care system in the United States. The takeover includes many of the centers of excellence—the university-based and -affiliated hospitals and clinics. Managed care has in reality come to mean managed billing that raises total costs, lowers payment for medical services, restricts medical services, undermines quality of care, and generates huge profits for the investors in these venture capital–driven enterprises.

Serious illness in ourselves or a loved one challenges all of us quite enough in life. We do not also need to be placed at risk by either the source of our care or the systems within which that care resides. Yet that is exactly what is happening. Efforts to counteract the profit margin–driven systems in U.S. health care are not anywhere near powerful enough to nullify the dangers to all of us that increase as the days, weeks, and months pass.

Over the last five years, as the health care cost debate grew in the political arena, large businesses discovered health care as a new frontier in which to make very large profits. The political debate became a wonderful smoke screen for the maneuvers of American and foreign corporations with venture capital monies to buy up, manage, and control the entire spectrum of health care—from materials, equipment, and medicinals to hospitals and licensed health care providers of all disciplines.

The Grim Realities of Managed Care

The process moves ahead swiftly as you read this paragraph. As advertised on buses, radio, through newspapers, magazines, and television, public relations messages tell us that the efforts of managed care are saving the public money. The reality is that the nonphysician executives of these organizations, as well as their major investors, are taking home millions of dollars, while the quality and appropriateness of care are being whittled away through a process that demands profit margins and marketing costs as high as $.30 out of each dollar.

Salaries of the CEOs of these systems reach millions of dollars per year, approaching and even occasionally exceeding the salaries of the CEOs of *Fortune* 500 corporations. In 1995 the salary of some HMO chief executive officers reached $4 to $6 million per year and were 107 to 227 percent higher than the average salary of CEOs in companies of similar size and performance in other industries. There is a real question in my mind about whether anyone ought to earn that kind of money from the misery and sickness of others.

At this time many of those covered by managed care systems (this includes HMOs) are actually owned, bought, and sold as patient populations—with the same indifference we are accustomed to from cattle and sheep buyers—by the various alphabet soup forms (HMOs,

PPOs, PHOs, etc.) of managed health care organizations and insurance companies with different brand names around the country.

Our society has always been one of merchants whose unrestrained buying, selling, and profit-generating activities in the eighteenth and nineteenth centuries had by the early part of the twentieth century to be restrained by government-imposed limitations: child labor laws, antitrust laws, fair trade laws, consumer protection laws. The free market that in fact works successfully in many places—in manufacturing, transportation, and distribution of products—is like a leech sucking the blood from weakened bodies of the ill. What should be a transfusion of comfort in difficult times now is more often than not just the opposite. Once again, Professor Rubin has an apt quote: "Health care is now a full-fledged industry: The actuary stands with the physician at the bedside."

The goods in health care, of course, are the services and materials needed to assist all of us in maintaining our health or recovering, when possible, from illness. Even dying is not excluded, for today more and more hospices are for-profit corporations. The quality of what is provided to us is relevant only in its relation to the bottom line of this juggernaut of managed care systems.

The "May I?" Game

Treating patients has become a paper- and telephone-encumbered game of "May I?" in which physicians find themselves less and less able to take action in treating or prescribing to their patients without first getting authorization from managed care company employees for each step, sometimes each medicine. This slows down the treatment process. It often infuriates and demoralizes physicians as well as patients. Patient care is put at risk, including the proper timing and sequencing of treatments.

The basic drive is to provide as little as possible for *as little as possible* while the traditional caring values of physicians and nurses are being eroded further. They are replaced by productivity quotients to which salaries and employment are linked and the linking of bonuses to successfully minimizing hospitalizations, procedures, and prescriptions. (Bonuses are for those shepherds who tend their sheep at minimal cost to the owners!) Productivity is measured on a monthly basis in these organizations; a few measure productivity on a weekly and daily basis. The physicians who remain in private practice are more and more linked to these systems if they want patients at all; they too are asked to adhere to contractual agreements in which access to patients is traded for significantly reduced fees of (by 1996–97) 30 to 60 percent.

What Can You Do?

Dealing with the direct and indirect costs of cancer treatment always presents challenges to your energy and ingenuity. Early on in your cancer odyssey you should review what resources you do have to help handle all the costs of treatment, care, and recovery. It will quickly become apparent whether or not you will need assistance and what kind of assistance you might need. Hospital social workers can often be of help as can the various cancer advocacy organizations. Special assistance for travel to major medical centers can be obtained through a consortium of major corporate jet aircraft on a space-available basis.

Many pharmaceutical companies have special programs to help defray the costs of certain medicines when such assistance is needed. They are called *reimbursement assistance programs*. The list changes regularly. It can be obtained from the American Pharmaceutical Association. Review the policy of your HMO or health insurance plan to be sure what it does and does not provide. If you think it should provide certain benefits that it does not offer, check with your state's health insurance commission office. Your state insurance commission may well have required-by-law regulations governing payment for second opinions, the legality of withholding information about innovative and new treatments, and the freedom to choose your own specialist based on experience and qualifications.

New national legislation will protect you from losing coverage when changing jobs or not getting coverage for your cancer because it is a preexisting condition. Report problems that are not resolved satisfactorily to your employer and the state insurance commission. Request that your employer offer only health insurance plans that are certified to have attained certain basic levels of quality assurance through certification by the National Commission on Quality Assurance. Don't be shy about seeking help from your local American Cancer Society and other local advocacy and community service organizations. If your employer has an open season allowing switches to new health insurance programs, never be pennywise and pound-foolish. As a cancer patient you need good medical coverage. You often get what you pay for with very low-cost plans.

Be wary and get consultation about accelerated death benefit or "viatical" insurance programs. There are more than 150 such "products" now, and they may track you down with solicitations even shortly after your diagnosis, sending shudders up your spine and piercing your hopeful heart with doubt. These companies will promise to buy your life insurance for 30 to 40 percent of its face value, giving you the cash to relieve your current needs in exchange for your signing over the benefits to them; thus 60 to 70 percent of your death benefits will not go to your survivors but to insurance companies, which consider these viatical settlements to be hot investments, according to the North American Securities Administrators Association. Selling out to their pressure may be very shortsighted, very ill-advised.

As you heal, become an advocate at the state and national level for regulations that push insurance companies, HMOs, and other managed care enterprises to provide information about the quality of what they really provide, especially for cancer patients. Become an advocate for limitations on the ability of insurance companies and managed care systems through their treatment and prescription review ("May I?") policies to practice medicine, an activity for which they are neither licensed nor regulated. Maintain yourself as an educated consumer, actively following the advice and care given to you, but only when it follows the best standards of care as you understand it. Remember that more and more doctors and nurses have literally become employees of managed care organizations or are held hostage by them in exchange for access to patients. As a result, we are all at risk not only for being denied access to cutting-edge treatments but even for not receiving responsibly delivered and complete care by yesterday's standards! In Appendix E of this book you will find resources that may be of help to you.

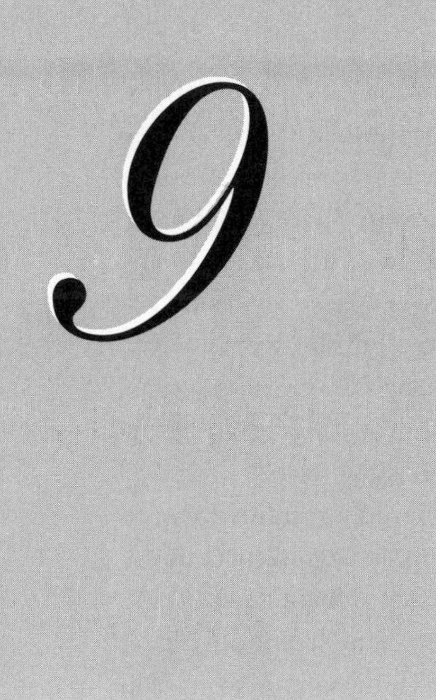

Controlling Your Tomorrows: Living with Uncertainty

MOST OF US, when we aren't sick, don't spend a lot of time thinking about the different parts of our bodies and how they function. Every part seems to be doing what it is supposed to do. If we are in good health, we don't think much about poor health. A patient once said to me: "I have had no sense of my own vulnerability." Many people feel this way, and it's healthy. Most people live with their illusions of certainty, of life stretching painlessly on to some distant time.

We often talk of teenagers having no sense of their mortality, but, we all, regardless of age or intellectual awareness or job, share at least some of that focus on today and maybe tomorrow. Only when we face significant physical limitations in old age or serious illness does the veil that hides the end from our emotional awareness slip from before our eyes. Then we see the horizon of our days. As a cancer survivor, you no longer can avoid thoughts about mortality. A cancer survivor lives always with doubts about tomorrow, with uncertainty. That is true when the diagnosis is new, it is true when the cancer is in remission, and it is true when you have been cancer free for years. Cancer, to steal the words of Samuel Johnson, "concentrates the mind wonderfully." Ignoring mortality doesn't make us immortal. You know that now better than ever before.

Our culture has trained most of us to feel, in the words of Dr. Balfour Mount, that "illness, wellness, life itself . . . certainly cure, food, health and happiness are part of our constitutional right. Serious illness is an affront: someone made a mistake here!"

Your experience with cancer has undoubtedly retrained you to a more honest view of life. You have, I hope, struggled successfully to accept the diagnosis of cancer, to educate yourself about and advocate for yourself within the medical system, seeking to meet the challenges of your illness rather than falling victim to it. You may still have moments when in dreams, daydreams, and fleeting thoughts you think your cancer diagnosis is an unreal horror story that will go away when you wake or shake the idea from your mind.

It is too late for that. You are no stranger to the ordeal of treatment. You have survived innumerable procedures, tests, and treatments, feeling proud that you have mastered, in your way, your suffering. You've both adapted to and modified the responses of family, friends, and community. You realize that you are now forever different from those who have never had cancer, even from those who have survived other life-threatening experiences.

During the diagnosis and beginning treatment of your illness these feelings of uncertainty and profound awareness of horizon weighed heavily on your consciousness, if only for brief periods of time. Then you became caught up in the physically and emotionally stormy period of the treatments themselves. Finally you are being granted some clarity, an apparent certainty: the sought-after goal is obtained—treatment is complete; your cancer is gone or in remission or under control. Which reality is yours depends on the kind of cancer you have, how soon you were diagnosed during its course, how advanced it was when discovered, the treatments received, the resilience of your body. Now, perhaps to your surprise, is when these feelings of "It can't be!" and awareness of a personal horizon weigh heavily again. Those of you whose cancer is in remission or under control will feel that your ordeal is over, that you've succeeded. Why don't you feel better?

You suddenly realize that you don't feel safe. Treatments have stopped: you feel that you no longer have anything to fight cancer with. At this moment you are confronted with mastering a new skill: living with uncertainty.

Living with Uncertainty

What to do? How to live? Can the old illusion of personal invulnerability be recaptured, the veil protecting you from the reality of a horizon be replaced? Weren't hope and hopefulness based on that sense of invulnerability? The illusion cannot be recaptured or the veil replaced. Memory does not allow that to happen.

As a cancer survivor you are forever a cancer patient—it is part of your life. In some ways, like a Vietnam War veteran, posttraumatic stress disorder (PTSD) is now part of your life: having gone through your cancer war(s), you have recorded those experiences using all your senses and emotions. Now a word heard or seen, an image experienced, a smell, a taste, a dream—any or all will bring back, unbidden, at unpredictable moments, experiences from your treatment that you would prefer to forget. The longer you are in remission, the fewer and less intense these PTSD experiences will be despite the reminders that occur at the regular checkups you have every month or every three, six, or twelve months. Hope must now grow from another root.

Living with uncertainty requires three actions on your part: (1) reexamining and appropriately rearranging your psychological defenses; (2) reflecting on your beliefs about life and then actively, broadly reengaging in life; (3) examining your sense of connectedness with all that is around you in the world and then maintaining that connectedness through rituals of thought as well as action. You need to engage in all three actions during the time your dependency on the medical system decreases. That decrease, or even loss of dependency, inevitably leaves you asking yourself "What now? When I was in active treatment, I was doing something. Now I am not doing anything to keep the cancer from returning. It snuck up on me once. Why won't it sneak back?" These thoughts send your anxiety soaring, often leaving you depressed.

Rebuilding Your Psychological Defenses

Rebuilding your psychological defenses goes hand in hand with letting go of your dependency on the medical system, its tests, test results, nurses, and doctors. Over the months of treatment your doctor, nurses, and others—even the procedures—became reassuring presences, voices telling you that you were fighting the cancer, doing your best to win the battle, choosing life. The health care system, its activities, and its members provided you with a structure within which your fears and other emotions could be contained. Now you find yourself standing on your own. Uneasy thoughts flood in: what does this ache mean? Why am I not hungry? Why am I so tired and sleeping poorly?

Negative thoughts often arise at this time as you compare yourself to others who do not have cancer. Sometimes the sense that you are a target for bad things floods in. The emotions of fear, uncertainty, anger, anxiety, and depression can wash over and even overwhelm you.

Understanding Psychological Defenses

The ways our minds function to help us cope with life—our thoughts and life events—are called our *psychological defenses*. Certain of them are universal. One of the ways we differ from one another, however, is our particular combination of these defenses, including our ways of using them.

All of us, every day in good health and bad, use denial, avoidance, sublimation, repression, suppression, rationalization, intellectualization, humor, satire, and dissociation. It is helpful for you to understand them. *Denial* means refusing to think about or focus on negative, upsetting things. *Avoidance* involves refusing to deal with difficult or upsetting things. *Sublimation* refers to intensely occupying yourself with other activities and chores. *Repression* is the process of unconsciously, automatically putting uncomfortable—fearful or angry—feelings out of reach of your conscious self. *Suppression* occurs when you consciously, deliberately decide not to think about a situation or an event. *Rationalization* means explaining things to yourself so you feel like they make sense, that they should indeed be the way they appear to be. *Intellectualization* occurs when you mobilize your logical self to synthesize observations and facts into conclusions that create a reality or illusion of understanding and through that understanding a sense of control. *Humor* consists of a state of mind that allows you to be distracted by perceiving experiences or events in a way that causes you to laugh or smile. *Satire* involves distracting yourself by using your mind to make fun of life experiences, even ones that are objectively rather grim. During cancer treatment you also probably rediscovered and used an old psychological defense from your early childhood to help yourself cope with frightening and painful experiences—*dissociation*. It means removing yourself, as in a dream or observer state, from the immediate, intimate experience of fear or pain or something extremely unpleasant or extremely unfamiliar.

Techniques for Recapturing Control

The need now is to analyze your particular psychological defense system. How did you cope with life before cancer? How did your mind help you deal with the ups and downs of life, including physical changes and changes in well-being and emotions?

Think about how you have been using these defenses and reconfigure them, using some more and some less, so that you reengage yourself in life free of the burdens and intrusions of treatment. This means avoiding, limiting, or ridding yourself of obsessive thoughts about your cancer's possible return. The psychological defenses of suppression, sublimation, and distraction through humor and satire are key techniques to use. Sometimes professional help (from a psychiatrist or psychologist or clinical nurse specialist trained in behavioral medicine) is required to deal with uncontrollable negative thoughts. Participation in an active cancer treatment or cancer survivor support group almost always helps a person develop and use the appropriate defenses.

Brief moments of fear will occur, but you will become more and more adept at pushing those fears away. As long as you accept and don't fight the normalcy of fearful thoughts, you will be able to control them and live with them as they occur. You will do so not only through use of the psychological defenses of suppression, sublimation, and humor but also through intellectualization and self-satire. Periods of diffuse anxiety and even depression are normal to experience after you have completed the first four to six months of treatment. This is part of the process of stepping out on the yellow brick road of uncertainty. Again, worries will decrease over time. That process of decreasing worries can be encouraged through a series (five to ten sessions) of empathetic, knowledgeable, professional assistance and/or by participation in a cancer support group led by an experienced mental health professional.

Redeveloping Trust in Your Body

As a cancer patient you sought help from the medical community to guard, protect, and recapture the health of your body. Part of letting go of dependency on that community involves incorporating as your own the knowledge about cancer, health, and self-care that you have learned from doctors and nurses. This is particularly important in the area of physical symptoms. You need to redevelop trust in your body's functioning. You need to allow yourself to receive, without excessive anxiety or fear, the messages your body sends out to you. Anxiety, fear, or ignoring of these messages blocks your ability to interpret them accurately and act, when called for, on them.

You will work to master the anxiety triggered by unexpected muscle cramps, twitches, bowel cramps, constipation or diarrhea, coughs, poor appetite, weakness, or unexpected pain. You must now assume responsibility for monitoring your body, for not ignoring symptoms. Any pattern of symptoms—any increased awareness of body functioning, any new sensation, any discomfort—lasting without a break or increasing in severity over five to fourteen days without a clear or obvious explanation such as catching a virus going around the community, requires you to check out these symptoms with your doctor. *Do not minimize symptoms.* Inquire whether or not a particular symptom is a cause for concern.

The challenge you face is that while containing your fears you must rid yourself of uncomfortable, even guilty uneasiness about bothering your doctor. Physical symptoms, as you well know, can include many things, such as loss of appetite, aversion to certain smells or tastes, poor energy or physical weakness, fever, flushing, various gastrointestinal symptoms, skin problems, localized or generalized pain, and headaches. You will master the ability to simultaneously track your physical symptoms—this does require a certain vigilance on your part—while putting them out of your mind, as hopefully you did before cancer, when unpleasant or different body feelings were fleeting and without pattern. (Symptoms that last or fall into patterns must be called to the attention of your physician.)

Matthew told the group: "I always had a bad stomach. I used to get stomach cramps as a kid in anticipation and fear of my father's anger. Now I have strange stomach feelings days after chemotherapy, especially when I smell certain foods. My doctor has helped me sort this out so that I'm not worrying every minute that something has gone wrong."

Of further help in interpreting and responding appropriately to symptoms is the intellectual exercise of reminding yourself of your understanding of your cancer, the organ systems it can affect, and the symptoms that can be produced by problems with those organ systems (heart, kidneys, lungs, bowels, brain, skin). Understandably you, like most people, would rather not do this thinking. But you are much better off in your mental and physical health if you make the effort to do so. If something, no matter how vague or difficult to define, seems wrong, check it out yourself and also have it checked out by the appropriate health professional. Often this will result in reassurance after further examinations or tests, but sometimes it will require a new course of action.

Either way, remember that you should continue your own treatments. You do this by building up your strength, working to adapt in any areas in which your self-image or functional capacities have been diminished through the illness or treatments, and continuously enhancing your body's capacities to heal and your mind's ability to monitor that healing. Such activities of mind become essential to reengaging in life.

Engaging in Life

When cancer treatments and the medical community no longer dominate your time and thoughts and other resources, you are free to recapture a personal sense of control beyond any you have had since your diagnosis. Dr. Peter Morgan put the choice this way: "You can let time go or orchestrate how you live." Just letting go is not a good decision. This is a time to redefine yourself and through that new self to reevaluate your priorities. You may find some aspects of your direction in life altered by this reexamination.

Rebecca, months after completion of all her treatments, was back to working thirty-five to forty hours a week—far less than she used to. Her job as a graphic artist included supervising an entire department with a large staff. In the evenings she was now finding herself totally drained, exhausted. A friend helped her consider her total situation: Perhaps the administrative responsibilities were draining her. Wouldn't her energy be used better and her work done better if she delegated much of the administrative responsibilities and increased her time in creative graphics work—something that was always joyful to her? She realized that this was a transition she should make for her own well-being.

Personal and work relationships change during the course of your treatments; they should now be reevaluated and readjusted. Relationships with important others such as spouses or children that were troubled before your diagnosis of cancer often stay fixed in that state while covered with a veneer of cooperation and support during the crisis of treatment. That veneer begins to fall away now. Since quality of life and optimal healing are your goals, your energy and time should now be directed toward resolving or improving those preexisting troubles.

Marie-Anne, relieved that her treatments were completed, found her husband similarly relieved. During her treatments he had been very attentive, considerate, patient, supportive, and warm toward her. Now that she was out of the woods, he showed his relief by returning to his behavior before her illness: impatient, manipulative, icy-aloof when he was displeased, refusing to disagree openly about anything—a control game of chronic guerrilla warfare that had marked their marriage for years.

Helping Family and Friends

For those of you who are fortunate enough not to have had significant troubles in relationships before your cancer diagnosis, family and friends need a new kind of attention. They too must readjust. As one individual correctly observed about the changes in use of time, energy, and activities undertaken, "My wife's life has been redefined by my illness." You may not need family and friends as much or in the same ways. They, too, need to evaluate the effects of the cancer experience on their lives and their perceptions. Some friends and acquaintances will have fallen away. You may wish to reinitiate contact with them, but you must be ruled by your newly acquired sense of priorities as well as your understanding of the preciousness of time and quality of life. On the other hand, you can, without guilt, send packing fallen away, fair-weather friends and acquaintances. The *shoulds* and *musts* of life are significantly diminished in importance.

It's damage control and review time. It's time to invest less cautiously in family, friends, career, and community. It's a time for relearning that your life schedule can be your own, that you no longer have to be as careful as you were during treatment to avoid stressors, infections, and demands on your energy. Having learned to truly value life, you begin to recapture thoughts of a future beyond the next day, allowing yourself the freedom and passionate intensity to define the future in terms of your needs and wishes.

Rachel, age fifty-two, was almost finished with her chemotherapy for breast cancer when she suffered a stroke. The stroke left her with some mild weakness of her left side, leg, and arm and difficulty finding words. Although steadily improving with the help of excellent physical and speech therapy, she became less and less motivated, more and more tearful, and withdrawn. Rachel responded very well to my treatments for depression: Her eyes were shining again; her speech was back to its normal energy and almost normal fluency; she was active and did not mind the cane she carried to help her when her left leg tired more quickly than the rest of her body. In reflecting on her situation, she told me: "I never in my life had any illnesses or sense of personal vulnerability. Now fears are always there. I deal with them by being active with friends, children, grandchildren, cooking—it's so creative for me—and shopping. At really bad moments I go to my bedroom and let the fears wash over me. If I don't fight them, it's over soon. And then I get up and go out again."

Pete, an accomplished surgeon, approached his own cancer as he would any surgical problem. He was out to make modern medicine help him beat the cancer. Treatments, he knew, would continue for some time. Then what? "What is life worth?" he asked. "What do I really care about and want? I already see that I want to practice medicine differently than I did before my cancer. I had no understanding of what it was like to be a patient. Most of all I want to spend a lot more time with my children and my wife."

Grieving for the Old and Accepting the New Self

Your treatments may well have aged or diminished you in some way: change in hair thickness, texture, color, or loss of hair; loss of muscle mass; ostomies and other possible altered physical parts; scars; chronic dry mouth; diminished energy and strength, etc. It is usual for them to do so. You may notice a somewhat different self at the end of the tunnel of treatment. You need to accept that different self. You may undergo some level of grieving for what you were physically before the cancer diagnosis.

Allowing yourself to grieve for the lost self frees you to be accepting and loving of the new self; this, in turn, allows others who care to respond to you more openly. Do not withdraw from others; or, if you have, correct that withdrawal. Do not get lost in concentrating on the past ("I had so much energy!") or worrying about current functioning ("I can no longer do the job!") or what others think ("Can I find any people who will value me?"). While paying attention to your own feelings and reactions, let yourself enjoy being with and observing the behavior of others and their feelings as expressed through their words as well as behavior. Increase your involvement with family, work, colleagues, and community.

Preparing Coping Strategies Now for Possible Future Challenges

Now is also a good moment to set aside a sufficient amount of time to consider and rehearse your behavior in case there should be a recurrence or relapse of your cancer. Educate yourself about the current treatment options if, in fact, that occurs. Let yourself become aware of nontraditional treatments too. Focus on learning about their positive and negative properties. (See Chapter 5 and Appendix E for recommended information sources.) Plan in advance who will help take care of you and what level of dependence you can have on others. Decide in this quiet, noncrisis moment what level of further treatments you will submit yourself to should they be needed.

Once you've gone through these steps and written down your decisions, put all this information away in a place where it can be retrieved if needed. When you have those normal moments of angst and worry, you will be free to use the healthy psychological defenses of rationalization and suppression by saying to yourself: "I've already planned for all of this. I know how to handle a relapse if it occurs. I can and will put that worry out of my mind, focusing my time and energy on the many things I can do for my quality of life and health."

Connectedness with the World Around You: Spirituality

Cancer shattered your illusion of personal invulnerability. Its onset does the same for all of us, presenting us with what Dr. Robert J. Lifton calls the "jarring awareness of the fact of death." Its diagnosis and the subsequent treatments create an exaggerated focus on body that in and of itself can become a possible health problem.

To our knowledge, we are the only species that, through self-awareness, organizes its existence and understanding of that existence with imagery as well as symbols representing life, death, and survival. Through this imagery we have, over time and in many forms, developed a unique awareness of life and death. How do we remain masters of that life and death imagery rather than live in terror of it? Through our contacts with death and the images we retain, how do we embrace life, fighting off fears of separation and loss of self? How do we maintain feelings of our personal integrity and of our connectedness with others? The answer lies in opening yourself up to spirituality. In his book *A Whole New Life,* Reynolds Price captures for me a dimension of this vision: "As I survived the black frustration of so many new forms of powerlessness, I partly learned to sit and attend, to watch and taste whatever . . . far more closely than I had in five decades."

Referring to the nonmaterial and intangible, *spirituality* differs from spiritualism because of its nonattachment to a particular philosophic or religious form of thought. That attachment is, on the other hand, the definition of *spiritualism.* The two words refer to the same general principles directing us to expand our awareness beyond immediate experience and beyond self.

After all, we occupy only one planet around only one sun, in only one small segment of only one of billions of galaxies. This awareness alone makes us wonder where any one of us, or the entire human race, fits. *Spirituality* anchors and answers, at least to some extent, this wondering and its attendant discomfort.

Spirituality means the process of celebration of life as you find it and as you can embrace it with all your senses, emotions, and reason. Striving for connectedness beyond the material with other people, other living things, and the world beyond yourself opens you to the possibility of moving beyond loss, separation, and grief. Connectedness opens you to a condition of mind untouched by suffering. You discover yourself linked to nature through thought, emotion, and energy.

Life Is a Gift

You experience life as a gift. You realize that the fairness of its length as we experience it is an issue of relevance to us as individuals but that it means little to the world beyond. The salvation of self in life and in death is found through acceptance of the limitations of our mortal selves combined with experience of our connectedness with all beyond ourselves. It is the nature of humans to engage in continuous efforts at maintaining that connectedness. Without such continuous efforts, both on our own and with others, we all get lost in focusing down on ourselves, overexperiencing every sensation and every fear. Our spirituality becomes obscured in a fog of anxiety and worries. We then live our remaining time in confusion and fear.

Developing your spiritual self allows you to free yourself from any odd feelings as a cancer patient—that you yourself are fine; your body has cancer. Your life has significance in the larger human context and in the unity of mankind with all nature. Your vital energies allow you to experience your connectedness with the world, earth, and sky through their energies. Opening up through your senses to life beyond your immediate physical self will revitalize you. This happens through a sense of being a part of the forces controlling life and death, rather than being the victim of these forces.

Attaining Communion with and Beyond Yourself

How do you accomplish this connectedness? In our incredibly material and ordered society, it is often difficult enough for adults to identify joyful activities, to rediscover the joy of spontaneous play where the sense of time is briefly lost. An openness to experiencing your vital energies as flowing to and with the vital energies of the world is basic to the approaches used in many forms of traditional healing as practiced in both the East and the West. Meditation, prayer, and ritual exercises such as tai chi and qi gong, especially when performed in a setting that allows you to be aware of the sun, sky, water, and living things such as other human beings and plants, encourages the capturing of that connectedness. Others succeed in directing senses, mind, and reason to the world beyond self through gardening and regular visits and walks in parks, the woods, or by the sea. If science links together views of life seen through the interlocking disciplines of biology, chemistry, and physics, the perspective of flowing, interconnected structures and energies that give form to our universe is far from fantastic.

Choose the means that work for you in seeking a communion beyond yourself. Especially, if you can, at least at times, include some other person or persons; then no sense of horizon will beat you down. You will indeed face your tomorrows without fear.

10 Terminal Illness and Dying

THIS IS A TOUGH CHAPTER to write and a tougher one to read and consider. But this book would not be honest without it. Rabbi Earl Grollman once said, "The greatest cause of death is living." This chapter then has material for all of us to consider. No one is exempt—not the young, not the perfectly healthy, not the purest and holiest among us. But as a cancer patient you particularly cannot avoid the thought of death, the fear that somehow your cancer may take control. You are stronger for facing the question, setting it aside if it is not relevant at this time, considering all your options if it is. All of that is better than avoiding the question altogether. Denial does not cure! Total denial of emotionally powerful realities does not help with quality of life or healing.

Being willing to explore your own understanding of death is just as important an issue for those cured and in remission as for those who have nothing more with which to fight the cancer. You need to use your remaining energies to reexamine your current feelings about the instructions for care, powers of attorney, living wills, and wills already completed by you, making changes as appropriate. You want to assure yourself that you, not the medical system or family members, have as much control as possible. This acknowledges the reality that much of the medical system and, not infrequently, family members have difficulty in releasing an ill person from their control.

You are needed more than ever to act as a comforting and supportive therapist to your loved ones and friends so that they can remain with you through your dying rather than self-protectively distancing themselves as so often happens. This is for your own good *and* theirs. There may be some special projects that you want to stay involved with as long as energy and life allow.

You want to make absolutely certain that as you are letting go of your capacity to function at higher levels you are assuring your control over issues involving your comfort (including pain management) and dignity (including appearance). Through such actions, and continued efforts at humor and satire, while your independence decreases and dependence on others increases, you will assure yourself of reasonable comfort, calm any fears of abandonment, and enhance, rather than diminish, your connectedness with others.

There is strength in facing a worst-case scenario, and it helps not only the patient and family but doctors and nurses as well. Yet the subject is too often avoided. A recent study noted that the subject of death and dying was never brought up in consultations by two-thirds of physicians ministering to seriously ill patients. That is not good medicine, and it is not surprising.

In today's medical education there is often no formal training in dealing with death and dying. Indeed the entire modern Western medical education system rests on the underlying theme that death is both an enemy and a failure. Beyond that, because of extraordinary advances in many fields of medicine over the last century, both layperson and physician tend to function as though all disease must be curable. It simply isn't. Pretending that it is serves the patient poorly and leads to distressing and unfortunate consequences.

Put another way, there is, unfortunately for patient and doctor, no training in how to recognize when to stop efforts at prolonging life, when to accept a reality that the doctor's role and responsibilities have been changed by the relentless progression of an illness. At some point a doctor needs to let go, to allow a peaceful, physically and emotionally pain-free death to occur. That is realistic, compassionate, and compelling but too often simply avoided by doctors and hospitals.

When you mix together lack of end-of-life training and the normal human tendency to avoid anything that is anxiety provoking, it is no wonder doctors have difficulty with this subject. Indeed seeing death as a failure not only guarantees avoidance of the subject when it should be dealt with but is also a significant contributing factor to an unintentional recurrent breaking of the physician's Hippocratic oath to "do no harm." Pain, tubes, and respirators do not signal success. In fact they do harm to the dignity and emotional well-being of patient and family, as well as to life itself in its fullest physical and spiritual meaning.

Harm *is* done when a doctor deceives. Seeing death as a failure drives many doctors, particularly oncologists, to push treatments beyond what is in the best interests of the patient's quality of life, and that is deception. When they treat the disease and not the patient—and that is an important distinction—breathing may be extended, a blood count may change, but life in its most meaningful definition is not made better or longer.

The Conspiracy of Silence

Thus guidance or even encouragement to explore the possibility of your death and your understanding of it will rarely come from physicians. Doctors, patients, and nurses, as well as family members, quietly engage in a conspiracy of silence as they all avoid the subject of death, suppressing and repressing their own fears. Each individual assumes, without testing this assumption on others, that others hold the same kind of fears. Dr. Sherwin B. Nuland describes in his book on dying the pretense needed to maintain the fiction: "The old scenario . . . we knew—she knew—we knew she knew—she knew we knew—and none of us would talk about it when we were all together." Those energies used to maintain the deception could be used much better to encourage healing and the quality of life, to help one another with feelings and coping strategies, to meet the need to be reassured about separation from loved ones, to clarify misunderstandings, to express caring and love. Deception simply never cures.

We all face two issues: dying, a process; and death, a state of being, or nonbeing. In our culture we tend both to confound and to confuse the two. Dying, a process, conjures up images and feelings associated with loss of control, physical pain, the emotional pain of separation from loved ones, anticipatory grieving, and fears of abandonment. Death conjures up fears of darkness, of at least a period of "disconnectedness" from others, as well as of the unknown. And for those embracing certain beliefs it generates images of a feared idea—purgatory or hell—or a state of peace or pleasure, heaven or nirvana, or simply honor or rest.

Death ideally is examined as a part of life during the course of your life. When cancer becomes an immediate issue in your life, death should be reflected on in some fashion: on your own but in interaction with the thoughts of others through the written word of the Bible, Koran, Bhagavad Gita, Cabala, other religious writings, poems, plays, essays; with others—religious counselors, family, friends, even some mental health professionals; or in support groups open to exploring end-of-life issues.

I'd never met her before. A middle-aged woman with metastatic cancer, she was forced by her husband and her oncologist, because of their concerns about her anxiety and depression, into allowing me to consult with her while she remained in the hospital. Within seconds after I had entered her room and introduced myself, she angrily, aggressively said to me: "I hope you're not going to make me talk about death and dying!"

One would think that considering and dealing with thoughts of death could not be avoided. But refusal to accept death as part of life is so powerful in our culture that it pervades even these situations:

- Your cancer has returned as an active, growing process (it may or may not have spread), and you are informed that no more traditional treatments are possible other than drugs being evaluated for their toxicity as well as possible effectiveness.
- No treatments of any kind have proven effective, and your total body is clearly in the process of failing despite some remaining ability to pursue interests, relationships, even work (a condition described as *terminal illness*).
- Your organ systems are failing, energy and strength are steadily ebbing away to a degree that your self-care is impaired significantly or totally, and even relating to other people is severely limited (the state of dying).

Terminal Illness

Terminal illness and dying are not the same stages of life. At the terminal illness point in your personal odyssey as at all other stages, you test whether what you feel or are told is really so. Bargaining with higher powers and health professionals, making wishes, and evoking imaginary forces involves many people, but for you it may or may not be part of the process of coming to terms with the reality of terminal illness. There is always some search for other options. These may include agreement to participate in experimental treatment protocols as well as increased openness to involvement with alternative, nontraditional treatments.

Others around you, as part of their caring and their own struggles with accepting the reality of your condition, will thrust on you information about treatments and approaches to care that they hope might change your terminal illness reality. Buffeted by your own emotions and wishes, plus those of others in your life, at some point you must grab again the reins of control over your life. You will make a decision about the quality of life you wish to have for whatever remains of life.

Remember that at this point, just as earlier, no doctor can tell you how long you have to live. Some will try, even pronouncing the time left with great authority. Others may feel pressured by you, or members of your family, to give a firm estimate of life expectancy. Those who do so are giving you no more than their guess about weeks or months based on a combination of their direct experience and summaries of mortality statistics from the medical literature. These often do not connect with the reality of any particular individual, namely yourself. In general I find such pronouncements unhelpful, even harmful, because they may actually be seen as an instruction. A very perceptive patient, Reynolds Price, once expressed this possibility very clearly as he wrote about his own experiences with cancer: "All my life I've tended to meet people's hopes. Predict my death and I'm liable to oblige. . . ."

Coming to terms with the reality of terminal illness makes it in many ways a time of sadness and regret because of the obvious reflections on the acts and events and interactions in life that may no longer be possible. The poignancy of this time, poetically summarized, involves reflections on "the good not done, the love not given, time torn off unused" ("Aubade," Philip Larkin). This reflection should include embracing your belief system about death, which may or may not have an organized religious context. It is the time when I believe the stages first articulated by Elisabeth Kübler-Ross in her book *On Death and Dying* has some relevance to the cancer patient: the partial denial as you go through a form of shock (dissociation) in response to the information about the status of your illness; the desire to deny that the information is true; the anger, sadness, and depressive symptoms of loss of motivation and partial withdrawal from others; the bargaining with doctors, healers, self, and "higher powers" intermingled with hope; the redefining of hope as you accept the reality of your condition. In reality, none of this occurs in fixed stages or exact sequences. Rather there is a roller coaster of internal events and emotions with much revisiting of issues that occurs over a time span varying from days to weeks to months.

This Is No Time for Passivity

Terminal illness is also a time (irony of ironies!) for vibrant action. You have many things to do in the time you have left. Those who participate in or wish to explore an organized religious belief system should do so, establishing and increasing those contacts at this time. This includes seeking pastoral counseling.

You need to inventory and reflect on the many things you have done to remain active and prolong your life, feeling pride and even joy in the efforts you have made. Since people do not want to die without cause, it is a time, through conversations with your doctors, to clarify your understanding of why your body has exceeded its ability to fight off the cancer and maintain its wholeness in the face of infection, toxicity, and failures of major organ systems. Such information makes acceptance of your condition easier. The result may be a transient reemergence of anger, rage, resentment, or even a dramatic, temporary decrease in your sense of clarity of thinking, of being where you are. Such psychological reactions are perfectly normal at this time.

Hopefully you have available to you a group setting in which your feelings can be expressed and where you can hear similar feelings expressed by others. Hopefully you will have family members and/or a spiritual counselor with whom you can talk openly. You may find that writing down your feelings, in addition to these other options or instead of them, will be extremely helpful to you.

Rashid, sent by his government to the National Cancer Institute for treatment of his advanced sarcoma, clearly understood after four months that the research protocol had only temporarily slowed the progression of his aggressive tumor. He missed his family, his village, the sounds, the smells, the food. In his loneliness, I encouraged him to return to reading of the Koran. We were also able to find a mullah from one of the local mosques who came to the hospital every week. The mullah worked with Rashid through the Koran and in Arabic, to encourage Rashid to feel strong in his decision to return home and to find comfort in that decision.

Dying

In dying, as in living, we can strive for the ideal. As in life, few, if any, of us actually attain that ideal: death coinciding with a gently, quietly evolving distancing of oneself from the elements of life and loved ones; death without pain, or if not, death with feelings of being numbed to life and therefore welcoming a respite, a cessation of physical and emotional pain, of troubles and worries; death with one's sense of dignity intact; death in safety—that is, in familiar, comfortable surroundings with friends and loved family members available and at least a few in attendance.

Dying is a time for farewells expressed in words and gestures. Your farewells to loved ones must be understood as not sending them away, for you need their presence until death, and they will need your presence after death through many good memories and reminders of loving times. In helping them with the farewells you should communicate to them, if at all possible, feelings of acceptance about what is happening and that you did your best to embrace life while it was yours. You can talk with them about their lives after your death. By doing so you help set the stage for the continuity that all humans seek. As one example of that continuity, consider the beautiful and wise words of Kirk Varnedoe during his eulogy for the National Gallery of Art's Gill Ravenel: "Through art I have come to know something . . . about the communal passed-on renewal of fleeting pleasures of the senses through well-handled objects, but perhaps more tellingly about the afterlife of unique human spirits in the things they make and love. This is culture's recompense for the fatalities of nature."

Paradoxically, you can remain in control by accepting the special kind of loss of control that death represents: its separation from possessions; separation from connections as known up until now with others and with the world; the loss of self-awareness. You are simultaneously free to believe, if that is your education, experience, and wish, in some form of human continuity beyond that of your failing biological self, in the ongoing spiritual existence of or connection with, at least through memories, those who continue on in life.

Hospice

I join many others in recommending the hospice system as a way of helping you to maintain control while dying. Hospice provides a support system and setting whose values and philosophy are directed at facilitating as much as possible for both individuals and their families the highest quality of life possible as they die—autonomy is respected; isolation is avoided; pain minimized; physical-social dignity supported; emotional, spiritual, and religious support are available to the level needed by each individual. There are hospices for children and for adults in many places in the United States. Some are freestanding, some associated with religious service organizations (many of these are nonsectarian in their operation), and some affiliated with hospitals and nursing homes. (Last year, about twenty-five hundred hospices in the United States cared for 360,000 patients, and about 80 percent of them stayed at home for their final weeks or months.)

Depending on the community and the circumstances, a residential or a home hospice will be appropriate. Home hospice services mean just that—bringing the services of hospice into the individual's home. Hospice services include nursing; home health aides; volunteer support for companionship, errands, homemaking, and transportation; pastoral care; infusion services for hydration, nutrition, pain, and other medications; physical therapy; necessary medical equipment; physician supervision; family support services; and twelve- to fifteen-month bereavement follow-up for spouses, parents, and siblings. Hospice services are supported by a mixture of Medicare funds and private donations; they are available to people of all socioeconomic levels. To be eligible for home or residential hospice services, a physician's letter is needed certifying that your degree of illness is such that in his/her opinion you have no more than six months of life remaining. Information about hospice can be obtained from the Hospice Foundation of America, the National Hospice Organization, or your local hospital's department of social services. (See Appendix E for addresses and telephone numbers.)

Assisted Suicide, "Release," and the Hemlock Society

"I have had enough of suffering and of being courageous; I'm tired of it all."

Over the years, in various combinations of words, different patients, especially those in chronic pain, have said this to me as a preamble to requesting that I assist them with their own demise. We need to reflect on several realities here.

Quietly, with respect, gentleness, and without public comment, physicians working with the dying have for decades facilitated the natural end-of-life process. Never are dramatic or elaborate techniques needed; never has it been considered murder or assisted suicide by those involved.

This reality differs greatly from the passionate push for physician-assisted suicide as dramatically forced into the public mind by Dr. Jack Kevorkian. I personally object very strongly to the phrase *physician-assisted suicide* as used so broadly by the medical profession, the media, and the courts. The essential issues have become clouded. Clearly, helping a chronically ill or terminally ill person to induce his or her own death is facilitating a suicide. Such action is a naive, negligent way to deal with problems of fatigue, pain, loneliness, depression, and the sense of life without meaning that so frequently accompany chronic and terminal illnesses. So much can be done to make life meaningful and to improve the quality of life. Unfortunately, relatively few physicians and nurses have received training that allows them to provide this care, nor is such care valued by the health insurance systems of our culture.

Quality of life during terminal illness and during the dying process should be paramount. Elements of concern include maintenance of self-respect when an individual is dealing with disfigurement, loss of control, control of pain, management of sleep, anxiety, and depression.

One's physical and social self are diminished in terminal illness and in dying. As part of the transition from life to death, the vibrant self is diminished and the conscious self may suffer. When the various forms of treatment to decrease and distract from that suffering as well as attempts at reformulating hope fail, we can ask is not "release" (a euphemism for facilitated dying) an ultimate privilege? In the United States, Canada, and Great Britain, the Hemlock Society's book *Final Exit* makes available to the public one source of information that allows individuals to act successfully on a decision to attain "release" from suffering by speeding up a process *that is already occurring*. Should death in such circumstances, when quality of life has become untenable for the individual and life is ebbing away, be sanctioned, even assisted, as it is in Holland and the Northern Territory of Australia? This question was presented to the U.S. Supreme Court on January 8, 1997. The court's decision, handed down in June of 1997, deferred dealing with physician-assisted suicide as an issue definable through constitutional law. It referred the issue back to each of the states to be dealt with through their laws. The decision guarantees continued public debate about assisted suicide in the United States.

My concern is that we do not have the checks and balances in the medical and social system, as exist in Holland, to review and help individuals with this decision. Nor, as I mentioned earlier, have most members of the medical community received training in care of the terminally ill and dying. I have found too many times over my twenty-five years of practicing medicine, while evaluating requests for "release," that the suffering could be diminished and the quality of life while dying enhanced through more skillful use of the many approaches to pain management, depression, anxiety, sleeplessness, and physical and social support.

Simply helping family members acknowledge to themselves and with the patient the reality of the dying process is of itself an important therapeutic action that, interestingly enough, results in a reembracing of life while it lasts. I would go so far as to declare that the majority of situations in which a patient requests that death be facilitated come about because of less than optimal care and less than optimal medical personnel(physician/nurse)–patient collaboration.

Since death is guaranteed to all of us, "release" should not be hurried, allowing for consultation with involved family and professionals. The suffering patient must collaborate in these consultations. Of course, if there truly are *no* means for controlling the experience of pain, of providing an acceptable quality of comfort and life to the dying individual, then "release" should be an ultimate, available freedom. My hope, however, is that we will move toward a better quality of care for the terminally ill and the dying.

I felt a momentary surprise.
Surprise that so beautiful a life should have closing
so like any other.
As if beauty can ever know a close.

Christy Brown

11 Hope: Today's Research and Tomorrow's Treatments

TOUGH TIMES shouldn't mean hopeless times. Hope, great expectations, and optimism can often be realistic even in the worst conditions since so much new is happening in so many areas of science that affect cancers and cancer patients. We are happily moving beyond the old limitations of cancer treatments that not-so-cynical consumer/patients described as following the simple formula of "slash, burn, and poison," referring to surgery, radiation, and chemotherapy. As primitive as all three were not long ago, they *did* save and prolong lives.

But the past is, indeed, only prologue. Much has changed in these three areas and in others, too. Collaboration among the medical specialties, engineering, physics, biochemistry, and computer sciences has increased and become more effective. Great advances flow in a steady stream, like healing waters from an unseen spring. Our current research is exciting, leading to the means and techniques for early detection and successful treatments. Today is not without hope. Tomorrow is even brighter.

In this chapter I will give you enough information to educate you generally about these changes and to encourage you to become an even greater participant on your own treatment team. I want to avoid overwhelming you with excessive medical details that cannot coherently be conveyed in a short chapter. In Appendix D, I provide more information about specific treatments, including possibly more scientific information than you may want to know about cancer treatment techniques and prevention. Not all of the information in the appendix will be related directly to your particular cancer, but I hope you will take heart in the fact that so much is happening. Realistic hope is helpful, indeed really essential, to the cancer patient.

Realistic hope arises from breakthroughs in every aspect of cancer prevention, detection, and treatment—in surgery, radiation, chemotherapy, organ transplantation, genetics, nutrition, and supportive care, including infection control. Each day we witness the coming together of many things: we understand the nature of various cancers better, and early detection is therefore more likely; new antitumor substances have been discovered, and we know better how to get them to cancerous cells while avoiding healthy ones. We are finding value in non-Western medicines and treatments. The FDA has significantly cut the time between testing and using new drugs. We know more than ever about preventing cancers by altering environmental conditions and seeking good nutrition. Techniques of surgery have vastly improved through the use of lasers, we know better than ever how to combine chemotherapy and surgery to diminish mortality rates, and those rates have been lowered at a phenomenal pace for some cancers. I intend to expand on some of these advances more fully here, but just remember that we live—and I use the word advisedly—in an exciting time beyond miracles, a time of great scientific strides.

I do not preach false hope, gimmicks as solutions, miracle "cures" of dubious value; nor do I deny the deadly possibilities of cancer.

But hope is important, faith in the future essential, and today both are truly solidly grounded on scientific and technological progress.

My excitement for tomorrow grows from what I see around me: that small gains in cancer research, without question, will be made each month, if not each day. Major gains may surprise us at any time.

Our understanding of cancers as more than a hundred different diseases, with the common characteristic of cells growing out of control, advances in leaps and bounds. Our ability to diagnose cancers grows explosively thanks to many new techniques. With them we understand even better what we observe.

As a result, supportive treatments and technologies—greatly improved over the last five years—contribute significantly to the quality of life of cancer patients and the ability of cancer therapeutics to be creative and innovative. These range from the mechanical to the molecular and include improved approaches to pain control and the increased use of mind-body stress management practices.

Discovery of new antitumor substances and productive experiments that expand our understanding of the metabolism and growth of cancer cells will continue ever more rapidly. Until recently one problem for patients was the tremendous delay between discovery of a new treatment and its widespread availability in the community, sometimes as long as eight to ten years. This terrible delay is also changing. In September 1995 the FDA proposed new regulations to allow for more rapid introduction of experimental treatments. They became the law in 1996.

We will inevitably know more about prevention and causes of cancer. Just as inevitably, cures for some cancers now considered untreatable will be found. Improved techniques of diagnosis already give us a head start on treatment once denied us until much later in the course of the disease. Treatment that is more precise will help avoid old ways of dealing with cancer, often damaging the body even as they did some good. The end of the twentieth century is—without question—an extraordinary time in cancer research and cancer therapeutics.

In short, we move toward more precisely targeted and more effective cancer therapies with fewer and fewer side effects, less poisonous to the body in general, with less damage to specific organ systems. The quality of healing and the quality of life for patients thus will be improved significantly.

Traditional medical sciences represent only one dimension of this exciting future. More and more attention is being paid to three other dimensions of the cancer challenge: (1) the importance of the environment and nutrition to prevention; (2) the importance of quality of life and its influence on healing; and (3) approaches to both prevention and therapeutics from other cultures and other healing traditions. A new openness to experiences and wisdom from all sources today encourages an enthusiasm to bring together the best of Western science with the best of the healing arts from everywhere. In combination, all of this creates the possibility for increasingly effective and increasingly humane treatments that may enhance longevity while improving quality of life.

Our capacity to treat the different forms of cancer has changed so much over the last forty years that what is normal today was science fiction in the 1950s. For example, we can put into long-term remission or cure more than 80 percent of the acute lymphocytic leukemias (and 50 percent of patients may now live a normal life span), Hodgkin's disease, testicular, and cervical cancers; we can sustain people who have metastatic disease with reasonable qualities of life for very long periods of time, now measured for some in spans of more than a decade. We can produce remissions for forms of cancer for which there once was no useful treatment.

Some of the exciting developments start with the traditional applications of surgery and radiation therapy but all used in more selective, less damaging ways. Others involve new diagnostic techniques, new follow-up and supportive treatments. Innovative, experimental treatments, early identification, and prevention create exciting news almost monthly. A number of these are described in Appendix D.

Surgery

Surgery is usually what people think of when you say *cancer*. It is an old and easily understood technique. The principle of cancer surgery was and still is very straightforward: locate and define the offending lesions, biopsy when possible to understand exactly what kind of tumor you are dealing with, then cut as completely as possible until you have reached healthy, cancer-free tissue. The hope has always been that the removal of the cancerous tissues would result in a long-term remission or a cure.

Today we understand more clearly than in the past which cancers respond best to this approach, including when the objective is limited to reducing the mass of visible tumor as just one step in treatment. We have better knowledge about what situations respond to combined treatments using radiation and/or chemotherapy and immunotherapy. We now know that the sequence for improved results for some cancers is radiation or chemotherapy before surgery and for other cancers radiation and chemo after the surgery.

The reality today is that cancerous tissues are more completely removed with much less trauma to the rest of the body and with fewer complications than in the past. There has also been an amazing decrease in mortality related to the operations themselves. Even some of the dramatic abdominal surgeries, once so devastating, so frightening, are far less so today. Cancer of the pancreas, for example, which had mortality rates of 25 percent or higher several years ago, today in the hands of experienced surgical teams has only 2 percent mortality. One of the most deadly forms of cancer, cancer of the head of the pancreas, until recently resulted in no survivors five years after diagnosis. Today 26 percent survive that long and longer.

You will also find great hope in how the world of cancer surgery over the last twenty years has changed considerably in the use of organ transplantation, new approaches to amputation and grafting, and the introduction of totally new technologies from other sciences.

New knowledge combined with new technologies, including many from other disciplines, brings many advances. People are better prepared for surgery. There is improved anesthesia, improved maintenance of body fluid balance, much less blood loss, improved infection control, more effective use of electric knives, lasers, and fiber-optic visualization systems for less traumatic surgery, and more attention to designing surgery that maintains the patient's abilities to function in all ways after surgery.

Neurosurgery presents one of the better examples of this melding of knowledge and technology. Appearing almost as a technique out of a science fiction movie, surgery on brain tumors in a few major medical centers now makes use of the fields of radiology (CAT scans and MRIs), physiology, laser physics, and computer science to precisely define the location, volume, and boundaries of tumors. Through a tiny hole, a laser can find a tumor the size of a large seed and burn it out.

Chemotherapy and Immunotherapy

The search for improved chemotherapies focuses on discovering new compounds that are even more effective in killing or arresting the growth and spread of cancer cells, which tend to grow and multiply more rapidly than normal cells. Improved use of the chemotherapies very much focuses on diminishing toxicities experienced by the body's healthy cells, reversing or "rescuing" normal tissues from toxic effects, and reducing the patient's experiences of side effects (fatigue, hair loss, mouth sores, nausea, and vomiting).

Much effort today is directed toward several other dimensions of treatment as well. Ways to improve the aggressiveness as well as the tumor-identifying and tumor-killing activity of the immune system, for example, already exist. Approaches range from vaccine development for the treatment of melanomas to using the cytokines, specific products of immune cells, as therapeutic agents. These treatments were pure fantasy not so many years ago. Immunotherapy, for selected patients, is now combined with chemotherapy to enhance the cancer-killing effectiveness of both forms of treatment. New techniques in chemotherapy administration focus on delivering as much as possible to the cancer itself and as little as possible to noncancerous tissue.

Aside from the chemotherapy agents, the most commonly used systemic antitumor agents are various hormones or hormone-production blocking agents. Their usefulness derives from the role hormones play in maintaining the health of certain kinds of cancer cells (some forms of breast and prostate cancer) or in modifying immune system functioning. In the former situation, treatment is usually directed toward reducing the amount of estrogen or testosterone in the system when cancer cells are known to be estrogen or testosterone dependent for growth. Every year our understanding of how to use hormones as well as hormone-blocking agents in cancer treatment improves.

Radiation Therapies

For over a hundred years we have known that radiation in certain doses is toxic to cells and to organisms. The general purpose of radiation therapy is to send discrete bursts of high-energy particles in a path so focused that it only kills cancer cells. The ability to do just this with minimal damage to other tissues increases every year.

Radiation can both shrink tumor masses and kill rapidly dividing cancer cells. New techniques reduce undesirable side effects. New technologies allow more focused delivery of higher radiation doses to cancer cells. New chemicals exist that can be delivered to cancer cells specifically so that they are more sensitive than normal cells to the killing effects of radiation.

Radiation treatments are used in many ways. They can be used as primary treatment for certain tumors such as early cancer of the cervix, cancer of many sites in the head and neck, and some lymphomas. For more advanced cancers of the same types, radiation best serves as adjunctive treatment. Radiation therapy can be used to shrink tumors before they are removed surgically, increasing the success of surgery while decreasing its risk to the patient. Alone, or in combination with chemotherapy, radiation can improve the preservation of both organs (such as the liver or brain) and structures (such as the breast, jaw, vocal cords). The results often include reduced disfigurement, improved function, and improved capacity to be out in public, retaining patients' employment, family, and social functions. Radiation can be one of the most successful treatments for the pain resulting from metastatic cancer to the bones. It also can result in improved neurologic and cognitive function for tumors impinging on nerves or the brain. These are summarized in Appendix D.

Improved techniques and planning for radiation therapy are significantly directed toward preventing or at least minimizing side effects. The ability to use radiotherapies with minimal damage to other tissues increases every year. Consequently, the number of individuals suffering from long-term radiation therapy side effects as well as dose-related side effects such as radiation fibrosis and osteoradionecrosis (both of which produce chronic pain) decreases every year. Collaboration of specially trained physicians called *radiation oncologists* with medical physicists and technicians known as *dosimetrists* is essential for these improved treatments. The use of computers and modern imaging (CAT scans, MRIs) techniques has enhanced that collaboration, and computer-generated three-dimensional images of the tissues or organ system targeted permits sophisticated treatment planning. The final result allows better targeting of tumors for maximum killing of tumor cells combined with maximum protection of critical structures and healthy tissues.

Treatments for Improved Quality of Life and Health

At the practical level the greatest contribution to patients, their immediate family members, their doctors and nurses came about through the creation of different forms of central venous access catheters that can be implanted through minor surgery. Their invention and use eliminates the problem of frequent venipunctures that can destroy blood veins. These catheters allow greater degrees of freedom for patients, more movement about the community, more clinic and home versus hospital care, including chemotherapy, transfusion, and hyperalimentation. Implantable catheters dramatically changed the practice of modern oncology, contributing significantly to improved quality of life.

Many other medical devices advance cancer care. Miniaturized mechanical devices with tiny computer-driven pumps can now be carried in a pouch or worn on a belt for continuous chemotherapy infusions or for continuous administration of pain medications. New drug delivery systems now exist that allow for hormone replacement through skin implants. Skin patch drug delivery systems for pain can stay in place for as long as three days. Artificial kidneys, peritoneal dialysis devices, even artificial lungs continue to improve, for temporary use, sustaining people in life while injured organs recover their function or transplants become available.

Nausea and vomiting, especially in reaction to chemotherapy, presented a tremendous source of anxiety, including a psychologically based condition of anticipatory nausea and vomiting, for cancer patients over the years. Newly developed medicines help millions of people undergoing chemotherapy reduce this misery.

For special forms of pain many new products exist. These include controlled-release pills, better pain-relieving creams and lotions, and special mouthwashes and gels. The impact of the loss of the ability to produce saliva or tears is diminished through the development of special gels and sprays. Research continues on different ways to control pain as well as mouth, intestinal, genital, and urinary tract problems.

The most extraordinary contributions from the world of molecular biology are the genetically engineered natural substances that are now given to produce needed increases in blood cells: red blood cells for oxygen; white blood cells to fight off infection and kill tumor cells; platelets to help stop bleeding. These substances have reduced considerably the need for blood transfusions, especially of white blood cells and platelets. This in turn allows much more aggressive, more effective use of chemotherapeutic agents. Both recovery time and quality of life are improved through the use of these new medicines. Many a life has already been saved. Many more will be.

Finally, as you know from earlier chapters, I consider mind-body techniques—from improved capacity to relax and modulate one's physical and emotional responses to identifying stressors to self-hypnosis skills—highly useful treatment techniques. Knowledge of them and their use is ancient but only now becoming widely accepted. They are also part of your hopeful future. These techniques can clearly help reduce or eliminate (without the use of medications) anticipatory nausea and vomiting.

Over time, improved management of stress responses not only alters the susceptibility to airborne infections such as colds or even tuberculosis but also increases your capacity to function and cope psychosocially with chronic disease. They can help immensely with fatigue, now recognized as a significant quality-of-life concern, that over 70 percent of cancer patients endure. Mastering these relaxation-response stress identification and management techniques represents not just the past and present but also the future in cancer treatment as much as advances in surgery, radiation, and chemotherapy.

So there is much to be hopeful about, much to encourage you in even the most difficult of times. Being passive doesn't help. Search for what can make your every day as good as it can be—as full, as caring, as comforting as science and you, the ultimate team, can make it. Enhanced quality of life along with increased survivorship represent, as we approach the year 2000, the treatment goals at the cutting edge.

12 Checklists and Reminders for Survivorship

EVEN WHEN WE KNOW the things we should do, even when we know what is in our own best interest, we often don't find time or focus to follow through. That is true when we are young and well; it is also true when we are neither one nor the other. When you are a cancer patient or family, the situation is no different, although doing what should be done is more important than ever.

I've discovered from patients that making checklists helps. The simple process of producing them seems to reinforce following through on good intentions. When we assign ourselves tasks, think about them, write them down, and then put them on our refrigerator door or on the dashboard of our car, we glance at them, absorb them even without meaning to do so. Those quiet reminders can be surprisingly helpful as we move around. This is the reason that I end this book with a checklist for survivorship, lightened up with a few quotes that I like and hope you will like, too.

The lists are organized in part as my chapters are, but clearly some flow over into other sections. You will, I hope, use these checklists to assist you in making use of what I have shared in this book. They are not commandments chipped in stone. Use what you can. They are simply recommendations you can build on with your own checklists for survivorship. My thoughts are with you.

Listen, Learn, and Live

"You can let time go or orchestrate how you live."

Peter J. Morgan, M.D.

- ☐ Strive to control your own future, your life, to the best of your ability.
- ☐ Don't wait to be fixed.
- ☐ Participate in your own healing.
- ☐ Think of yourself as a member of your own medical team.
- ☐ Examine your fears, honestly laying them out for yourself. This is the first step toward mastering fear.
- ☐ Try to understand all that is happening. Educate yourself as necessary.
- ☐ Increase your personal skills through that education.
- ☐ Learn how to make your health care providers listen to you.
- ☐ Remember that your ultimate goal must be to lead the highest quality of life, by *your* standards, as possible.

The Fountain of Life Within You

- ☐ Remember that your body is continuously trying to heal itself.

- ☐ Understand as much as you can about your form of cancer.
- ☐ Don't think or ask "How long do I have?" Nobody knows.
- ☐ Reorder your priorities.
- ☐ Modify your lifestyle for your circumstances.

Clinic, Hospital, and Health Professionals

"He had had much experience of physicians and said, 'The only way to keep your health is to eat what you don't want, drink what you don't like, and do what you'd rather not.'"

Mark Twain

- ☐ Listening, observing, asking—all result in learning.
- ☐ Be an advocate for yourself.
- ☐ You need allies in your health care, particularly your primary-care physician, your nurse practitioner, or your physician's assistant.
- ☐ Keep your oncologist and your primary-care physician informed of your suffering from illness or treatments, as well as generally aware of other life problems that are currently challenging you.
- ☐ Make the medical system give you the information you feel you need to participate in your own care and healing. Insist on it!
- ☐ Get a second opinion. Sometimes you'll need a third, even a fourth, but please don't shop for the opinion you want to hear.
- ☐ Get further opinions when you feel you want them about tests as well as treatments. (You cannot be legally blocked by anyone from obtaining this information.)

- [ ] Ask questions (over and over if necessary) to clarify and/or reassure yourself about your understanding of what is happening or of what you are told.
- [ ] Check out the physician's experience with and frequency of performing complicated procedures before submitting yourself to them.
- [ ] Keep a pad of paper or a small notebook and pen/pencil with you.
- [ ] Write everything down.
- [ ] Have a pruned-down copy of your medical records in your possession. Keep written statements about your diagnosis and the basis for it, as well as hospital discharge summaries and written reports of x-rays, CAT and bone scans, MRIs, etc.
- [ ] Have your own master list of your drug allergies or unusual sensitivities.
- [ ] Keep a list of all medications prescribed for you.
- [ ] Add in the over-the-counter, homeopathic, naturopathic, or herbal medicines you take.
- [ ] Understand the major side effects of medications you are taking, remembering to keep your medical team informed of any side effects you experience.

Increasing Your Healing Skills

In those green-pastured mountains
of Fotta-fa-Zee
everybody feels fine
at a hundred and three
'cause the air that they breathe
is potassium-free
and because they chew nuts
from the Tutt-a Tutt Tree.

This gives strength to their teeth,
it gives length to their hair,
and they live without doctors,
with nary a care.

Dr. Seuss, You're Only Old Once!

- ☐ Health maintenance remains your job.
- ☐ Develop your skills in responding to stress. (Those skills involve both body and mind.)
- ☐ Learn to be patient.
- ☐ Maintain your grooming and dress—they help your morale and that of those around you.
- ☐ Keep to a regular day-night cycle if you possibly can.
- ☐ Maintain your interests and activities.
- ☐ Exercise regularly if you can.
- ☐ Pace yourself in work and play.
- ☐ Have a sense of humor and an appreciation of satire.
- ☐ Maintain your dental health and oral hygiene.
- ☐ When your immunity is down as the result of treatments, avoid crowded places: movie houses, concerts, sporting events, public transportation during rush hour, airplanes.
- ☐ If you can't avoid such situations when your immunity is down, wear a mask.
- ☐ When immunosuppressed, peel your fruit, steam your vegetables, and avoid salads.
- ☐ Do not sleep next to anyone, adult or child, when he or she is ill with a cold or upper respiratory infection.
- ☐ Use your imagination in a positive way to prepare for medical procedures and surgeries.
- ☐ Maintain proper nutrition with proper supplemental vitamin intake.
- ☐ Avoid, or at least minimize, your exposure to known physical toxins, including alcohol and tobacco.
- ☐ Maintain physical and emotional connections with others.

- ☐ Seek ways of giving yourself joyful moments and engage in them! (Only in joyful moments do we find the absence of fear, the absence of worry.)
- ☐ Learn to recognize anxiety and depressive states that exceed several days' duration.
- ☐ Make your immediate physical surroundings, as well as nearby space, as compatible as possible—temperature, sounds, density of people, etc.
- ☐ Meet, as much as possible, your basic economic and material needs, reaching out to family, friends, and community when support will help.
- ☐ A sense of spirituality is important. Develop a relatively continuous way to have the experience of, as well as sense of connectedness to, life beyond your own.
- ☐ Do not suffer in silence.
- ☐ Consider biofeedback and training in breathing and musculoskeletal relaxation techniques.
- ☐ Consider yoga, tai chi, and qi gong, personal trainers, physical therapists, Alexander and Feldenkrais practitioners if they are available and you can afford them.
- ☐ Consider the involvement of clergy counselors and behavioral health providers (properly credentialed psychiatrists, psychologists, clinical nurse practitioners, and social workers).
- ☐ Join a cancer support group and stick with it for at least twelve months.

Taking Control of Your Pain

"I was plunged into degrees of pain and . . . realistic depression that produced a dangerously passive state.

In that psychic bog of helplessness . . .
I was transfixed . . . by . . .
my undiminished physical pain."

Reynolds Price

- ☐ Decide what kind of good patient you should be. "Good" patients who do exactly what they are told, do not question, do not suggest, do not demand often suffer more and tend not to survive as long as feisty self-advocates. Being a bad patient—one who questions and demands reasonably—is really being a good patient.
- ☐ Don't let any health professional shrug off or minimize your feelings of pain as though they are not real or don't exist.
- ☐ Understand the usefulness of pain as information about your body.
- ☐ Learn how to communicate to health professionals about your pain.
- ☐ Learn about the many different ways—from medications to self-care, massage, and mind-body techniques—that control and modify the experience of pain.
- ☐ Pay attention to and get assistance with the fatigue and depression that always accompany chronic pain.
- ☐ Sleep disorders require treatment.
- ☐ Don't let pain isolate you from others.
- ☐ Massage and gentle forms of ritualized exercise like tai chi or qi gong or yoga help you live with chronic pain.
- ☐ Acupuncture helps with some forms of pain. It can do no harm, other than to your pocketbook! (Some insurance and managed care companies now cover acupuncture costs.)
- ☐ Use psychological techniques such as distraction and self-hypnosis as much as possible for managing and living with pain.

- ☐ Combining different medications under the guidance of an expert often gives the best pain relief.
- ☐ Alcohol use and chronic pain do not go together.
- ☐ Narcotics need to be understood and used intelligently.
- ☐ Always use pain medications when your pain is at its lowest level.
- ☐ Avoid confusion about pain medications by using pill boxes with dose compartments.
- ☐ Don't use powerful pain medication directly from the bottle, especially if nighttime use is needed.
- ☐ Work with your doctor and nurse to find the best combination and form of pain medications for you.
- ☐ If invasive pain control techniques—injections, nerve blocks, nerve ablation surgery—are suggested, get a second opinion before you do any of them.
- ☐ Third opinions by totally independent experts should be obtained if surgical interventions are recommended that involve the destruction of tissue.

Nontraditional Treatments

- ☐ No alternative treatment cures or prevents any of the cancers.
- ☐ Beware of those who overpromise.
- ☐ Beware of those who demand large amounts of money up front.
- ☐ Remember that *natural* or *herbal* does not necessarily mean harmless or helpful.
- ☐ Some alternative treatments, such as massage and acupuncture, may improve your healing capacity.
- ☐ Used thoughtfully, and in a complementary fashion to your traditional treatments and to proper self-care, a

number of alternative practices can improve your sense of well-being as well as your sense of control and hopefulness.

Family and Friends

". . . you and I were there and all the world."

Christy Brown

- ☐ Remember that your cancer touches the lives and thoughts of everyone in your family and friendship network.
- ☐ Keep control, but don't keep secrets.
- ☐ Children of all ages need to be kept properly informed at an appropriate level.
- ☐ Have family-friendship meetings in person, by telephone, by letters, and by e-mail to help others help you and understand your feelings and needs.
- ☐ Ask for help and even assign helpful tasks.
- ☐ Serious preexisting family problems need the assistance of behavioral health professionals (counselors) when cancer becomes an added stress.
- ☐ Help family and friends make use of appropriate advocacy groups and information sources: see Appendix C and Appendix E for this information.

Community and Work

- ☐ Keep working if you can.
- ☐ Adjust the intensity of work to your energy level and healing needs.

- ☐ If you were looking for an excuse to change or leave your work, use your cancer diagnosis as a disguised opportunity to make the desired change.
- ☐ Confront fear, rejection, and prejudice in the workplace if you encounter them.
- ☐ Use the various cancer advocacy organizations to assist you as needed.
- ☐ Be aware of and make use of the federal and state laws that protect your rights to sick leave, family leave, and job protection.

The Costs of Treatment and Insurance

- ☐ Understand the direct and indirect costs of your care.
- ☐ Determine what is covered by your insurance.
- ☐ Investigate available helpful community resources.
- ☐ Learn how to use them.
- ☐ Be *very* careful about viatical (accelerated death benefit) insurance offers in exchange for cash on any regular life insurance you may have: it's a for-profit business feeding on your financial anxieties during illness at the expense of you and your family.
- ☐ Quality treatment should be based on standards of experienced health professionals, *not* managed care, HMO, or other insurance organizations. Insurance companies are not health professionals. HMOs are frequently run as a business first and a health provider second. Don't be pushed around by them. Fight back!
- ☐ Seek legal assistance whenever you feel you may be getting less than the best treatments or medications for reasons of cost. Check to see if laws to protect you have been passed recently.
- ☐ Be vigilant concerning your care.

Living with Uncertainty

"Once cancer strikes, it is always stalking."
Sam Donaldson, ABC *News*

"So this is my life. How can I make the best of it?"
Diane Beaudin Sheahan

"Sleep . . . Balm of hurt minds,
great nature's second course,
Chief nourisher in life's feast."
William Shakespeare

- ☐ Reexamine your ways of coping.
- ☐ Use humor and satire to help distance yourself from frightening situations.
- ☐ Redevelop trust in your body, knowing what changes can be ignored and which ones need attention.
- ☐ Proper rest and sleep are vital. Make sure you get both.
- ☐ Consider your understanding and beliefs about death; avoiding doing so gives death power over you.
- ☐ Reengage as intensely as possible in your activities of life.
- ☐ Treasure and attend to your relationships.
- ☐ Relate every day in some way to people and other living things beyond yourself.
- ☐ Seek and cultivate a spiritual dimension to your daily existence.

Terminal Illness and Dying

"Life does not cease to be funny when people die, any more than it ceases to be serious when people laugh."
George Bernard Shaw

"The long habit of living indisposeth us for dying."

Thomas Browne

**"Death on a grand scale does not bother us . . .
personal death is an indelicacy.
[Yet] dying is, after all, the most ancient and
fundamental of biologic functions."**

Lewis Thomas

- ☐ If your illness has become terminal, make plans—a living will, durable power of attorney, a will, other instructions—then put them aside and live to your fullest for as long as you can.
- ☐ Examine again your understanding of death.
- ☐ Looking back into your childhood, ask yourself what you believe and what you want to believe about death.
- ☐ Ask yourself whether you are afraid of death or merely of dying.
- ☐ Plan ahead and leave good instructions so that you will not be left in pain or alone in final days. Discuss your wishes far in advance with your primary-care physician.
- ☐ Consider home or residential hospice care.
- ☐ Give those you love permission to go on living and, if you have a spouse, to have new relationships after your death. Someday we are all going to be someone's memory.

Future Hope in Prevention and Treatment

- ☐ Be comforted that efforts at prevention of cancer, early identification, and the many forms of supportive care and treatment advance significantly every year.

- ☐ Every several months, check the National Cancer Institute's Physicians' Data Query system for developments in the treatment of your particular kind of cancer.
- ☐ Subscribe to responsible commercial information sources such as *Coping* magazine and check regularly with your local cancer advocacy organization about new developments in treatment and supportive care.
- ☐ Devote some of your time to being an advocate in your community for the care and treatment of cancer patients—child, adolescent, or adult.
- ☐ Support, as well as you can and in any way you can, government and private efforts in cancer research.

A Note About the Appendixes

THERE IS SO MUCH going on in cancer treatment that it would have been easy to overload this book. I have tried to avoid that, treating the chapters just as I would one of my seminars, dealing mostly with questions people have and would like to ask. But I wanted a way to provide more material that is important but not universally relevant. That is why these appendixes are here.

Not all the material that follows will likely be of interest to you. Some is scientific background information—some people like to know it, and others could not care less. Some is specific to a particular kind of cancer and may be of no interest to people who do not have that precise condition. Information on alternative treatments, for example, may be of importance to a small but growing percentage of readers and rejected out of hand by others. There may be only one or two resources you care about.

You can easily lose yourself in a forest of resources for cancer patients and their families, needlessly spending energy in first finding and then choosing from lists and recommendations. Once again, I have tried to do here what I would do in a face-to-face meeting at one of my seminars—keep things simple even while trying to anticipate a variety of needs, limiting my recommendations to what I think will be of interest and help.

I hope you will simply treat this material as you would a travel or nature guide, seeking out what you want to know when you need it, looking for confirmation or expansion of ideas you have found in the body of the book, skipping what is of no relevance to your condition, thoughts, or concerns.

Appendix A: Pain Medication

PAIN, AS I NOTED in Chapter 4, is something that we feel both physically and emotionally. From common and lifelong experience, we should all easily understand that. For even in good health, a headache or a toothache not only hurts but makes us jumpy and difficult. Cramps or a twisted ankle often make us miserable, affecting how we feel and how we interact with others. Those pains, with an aspirin, ice, or rest, are gone in a matter of hours or a few days.

But things are more complicated for a cancer patient, who inevitably suffers repeated experiences with pain in a context of significant threat to self. The goal of treatment is to eliminate, whenever possible, the causes of that pain. When treatment is most successful, there is, of course, a complete, if gradual, end to the pain. But some pain just can't be eliminated.

Pain that is chronic—that won't go away—requires three approaches for successful management: (1) diminishing the feelings of pain, (2) increasing the ability to divert attention from the pain, and (3) diminishing the fatigue, sleep problems, anxiety, and depression that often accompany chronic pain.

My hope is that you will keep in mind the importance of understanding and communicating the nature of your particular pain; then, that you will make use of the techniques of proper breathing and related relaxation skills to ease that pain.

It is important to exercise appropriately and to use massage, ice, and heat where they provide relief for your specific pain. For some, acupuncture is also effective in dealing with pain.

Finally, I believe that *you must always be an active member of your treatment team*, communicating to your doctor-nurse team as precisely as possible what you are enduring. That is an important basic skill for successful pain management. Your description does not have to be complicated, but it does help if it is rather specific.

For this reason, several simple, straightforward, widely used pain intensity and distress scales are printed here. Familiarize yourself with them and use them as often as you need them. When you score your pain on these scales above level 5, it indicates pain that substantially interferes with your quality of life. Pain from level 7 through level 10 should tell your physician that you have pain so severe that it interferes with your capacity to function.

A single treatment approach is almost never sufficient for chronic pain. Various forms of radiation therapy, for example, are the most effective treatment for bone pain, pain from cancer-produced fractures, and tumor-induced spinal cord compression. But the use of medications is a vitally important approach to pain management and the most common way that cancer patients deal with pain. Medications help not only with the pain itself but also with secondary reactions such as sleeplessness and irritability and depression.

Medications for pain fall into several categories, analgesics being the most common. They decrease the feeling of pain, and they can be administered in widely different ways: by application to the skin; by mouth in pill or liquid form; by nasal spray; by cross-skin absorption (transdermal) systems; by rectal suppositories; by injection into the skin or muscles; intravenously; and by catheter into the cerebrospinal fluid. The selection of method depends on many factors: where the pain is and is coming from, how severe it is, and how

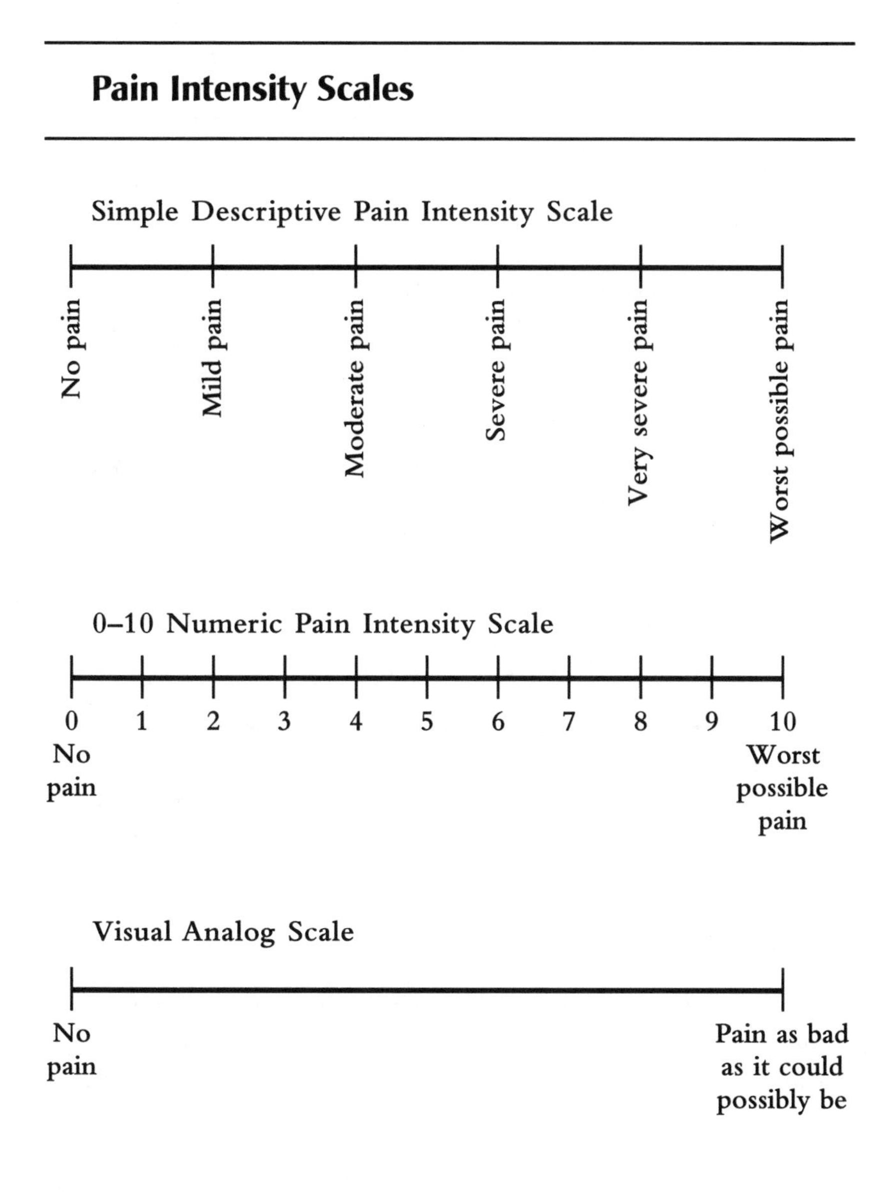

the medications selected can be best absorbed. Other considerations include the speed of pain relief desired and possible limiting factors to the method of administration such as mouth sores or nausea caused by chemotherapy.

Other medications used to treat pain function quite differently from the analgesics, but often they must be used with the analgesics

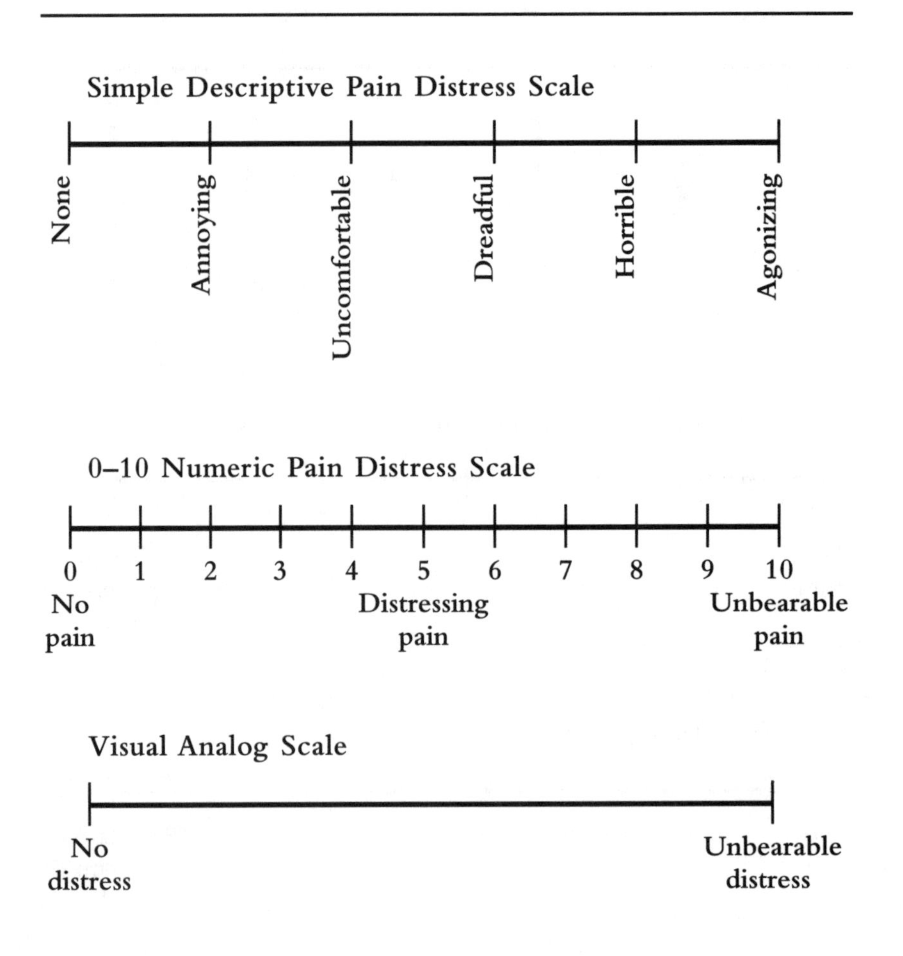

if the best possible pain relief and tolerance are to be achieved. Some of these medications alter your pain threshold—that is, your ability to tolerate pain; others relax the tension of skeletal muscles; some increase the effectiveness of the analgesics; others treat the conditions that arise in reaction to the pain experience such as anxiety, sleeplessness, and depression.

Analgesics

Topical

The three most readily available analgesics that can be applied to the skin provide reduced pain sensation only in the area to which they are applied. They give what is called *topical pain relief.* These include Fluori-methane (a skin-freezing spray), which gives only very brief relief; capsaicin (Zostrix-HP), a cream that can help with surface peripheral nerve pain (neuralgias), surface, or arthritic pain; and Emlin cream for local anesthesia for use before painful, skin-puncturing procedures.

Nonsteroidal Analgesics

This group of pain medications includes many that can be obtained in low doses without prescription. That does not mean you can take them without danger. Indeed, it is quite possible that more serious problems with the liver and kidneys, adding significantly to any pre-existing serious medical problems, are caused by the ever-popular acetaminophen (often known under one of its brand names, Tylenol) than by all the much-maligned narcotics combined. Some of these medications reduce fever or inflammation or both.

Table 1

Aspirin*	Indocin
Anacin*	Lodine
Ascriptin*	Meclomen
Aspergum*	Medipren*
Advil*	Motrin*
Aleve*	Naprosyn*
Anaprox*	Nuprin*
Ansaid	Orudis*
Bufferin*	Ponstel
Clinoril	Relafen
Daypro	Tolectin
Ecotrin*	Toradol
Empirin*	Trilisate
Excedrin*	Voltaren
Ibuprin*	

Table 1 gives a listing of some of the U.S. brand names. Different ones may in fact be the same drug, just packaged and named in distinctive fashion for commercial, trademark reasons. An asterisk indicates those available without prescription. Note that all of these medications can irritate the stomach. Some can produce gastrointestinal bleeding, some (the aspirin-based compounds) in high doses can produce systemic toxicity that is life threatening, and many can produce blood-clotting problems that make surgery much more dangerous.

The side effects of these medications can be reduced by dividing the daily dose, taking them with food and liquid and stomach-protecting substances. All of them can be used in combination with narcotics for pain relief if there are no drug allergies or other limiting factors present.

Steroids as Analgesics

Steroid medications such as prednisone, cortisone, and dexamethasone can through their powerful anti-inflammatory effects reduce the experience of pain. However, their systemic effects, particularly on the connective tissues and bone, as well as frequent altering effects on mood, energy, sleep cycle, and clarity of thinking, suggest cautious use. Because of these side effects, their long-term use for pain management is not ordinarily recommended.

Narcotic Analgesics

All narcotic medications require prescriptions in the United States. *They are remarkably safe medications for long-term use for the treatment of chronic pain.* They do, in subtle ways, blunt liveliness, leaving the patient rather "mellow." Some studies of long-term administration in animals indicate a possible mild reduction in the activity of the immune system; this effect has *not* been demonstrated in humans. Tolerance can develop to their pain-blocking effects, resulting in a need for increasing amounts of medication to obtain the same results. This form of tolerance, however, is not often seen in cancer patients with nonescalating chronic pain. Tolerance does develop—and that's good—to some of the undesirable side effects such as constipation and sedation, which lessen over time. These side effects tend to diminish the longer a particular dose of narcotic is maintained. Sudden cessation of narcotic use does result in withdrawal symptoms. These include sweating, chills, shaking, sugar craving, and loss of energy. Such symptoms are not life threatening; just awfully uncomfortable. We now have medications to minimize withdrawal symptoms should such help be needed. In very large doses morphine in particular produces depression of the activity of the breathing control centers in the brain. This effect has to be balanced against the sought-after pain-relieving effects of the drug. Proper pain management includes the physician authorizing

Table 2

Codeine	MSIR
Darvon	Nubain
Demerol	Oramorph
Dilaudid	Oxycontin
Dolophine(methadone)	Roxanol
Duragesic	Roxicodone
Levo-dromoran	Stadol
MS Contin	Talwin

the patient to use extra ("rescue") doses of narcotics for episodes of severe peaks of pain.

Narcotics consist of medications such as codeine, heroin, and morphine derived from the opium poppy. There are also laboratory-created narcotics that affect the brain in similar ways. They include propoxyphene (found in Darvon), pentazocine (found in Talwin and Talacen), methadone, meperidine (the active ingredient of Demerol), and fentanyl (the active substance in Duragesic skin patches).

Reactions to narcotics vary. Often more side effects of concern are experienced with the laboratory-created forms. Demerol in particular can result in confusion as well as hallucinations. Narcotic medications can be given as syrups, liquids, suppositories, pills, through transdermal skin patch delivery systems, injections, intravenously, and into the cerebrospinal fluid. Table 2 lists some of the more widely used narcotics.

All narcotics interact with other sedating substances, including alcohol. New pain medications that are nonaddicting yet block some of the opiate receptors in the brain, thereby making a patient feel less pain, are being developed. One of the newest of these, a medication called Ultram, although nonaddicting and often very effective, produces in some people unpleasant side effects such as alterations in the clarity of thinking, fatigue, and sometimes severe gastrointestinal discomfort or nausea.

Adjuvant Medications

These medications contribute enormously to the management of chronic pain. Indeed, their use in creative combinations has contributed to the greatest improvements in pain management during the final decades of this century. They do many useful things. Some help to quiet down irritable, inflamed nerves. Others raise the pain threshold. A group of these medications reduces muscle tension. Then there are the medications that reduce anxiety and tension, stimulating the brain in a way that counteracts the sedating effects of narcotics while increasing their effectiveness. They also improve sleep and decrease or eliminate depression.

Table 3 lists many of these very different medications by brand name. Selective explanations about them are in the following sections.

Antianxiety Agents

These medications, used carefully in combination with analgesics, often yield greater comfort than the analgesics alone. (They are used more in the evening than during the day to diminish the impact of sedating side effects.) The most rapidly acting of these medications, the benzodiazepines, are addicting. Some of them have useful secondary effects, reducing depression (Xanax), muscle tension (Valium), and the irritability of peripheral nerves (Klonopin). Some

Table 3

Ambien	Flexeril	Restoril
Ativan	Halcion	Risperdal
Baclofen	Haldol	Ritalin
Benadryl	Klonopin	Serax
Compazine	Lioresal	Serzone
Dalmane	Lithium	Soma
Depakote	Mexitil	Tegretol
Desyrel	Neurontin	Thorazine
Dexedrine	Pamelor	Tofranil
Dilantin	Paxil	Valium
Doral	Prozac	Xanax
Effexor	Remeron	Zoloft

medications in this family of chemicals are actually used as sleep-inducing substances. Most frequently used for anxiety are Ativan, Serax, Valium, and Xanax.

Anticonvulsants

This varied group consists of medications that tend to stabilize the transport of calcium across cell membranes. They have to be monitored carefully for clinical effects such as impaired coordination, sedation, and their effects on the bone marrow and liver function. For some of these medications we can combine our clinical observations with exact measurements of blood levels. Most commonly used today are Tegretol, Depakote, and Klonopin. Sometimes both lithium carbonate and Dilantin are included in this group.

A new medication called Neurontin (gabapentin) is currently being used by neurologists to help with pain syndromes.

Antidepressants

In *very low doses* some antidepressants such as Elavil apparently reduce the transmission of pain signals as they are carried from the spinal cord to the brain, hence reducing the perception of pain. Most antidepressants in my experience help improve the tolerance of chronic pain patients to their pain as well as improve their mood state and consequently their quality of life. Your physicians should work with you, when an antidepressant is recommended, to select one based not only on any past experiences you may have had with these substances but also on their known side effects. Side effects can include dry mouth, changes in bowel function, headaches, difficulty in focusing vision, weight gain or weight loss, changes in blood pressure, and changes in cardiac conduction.

There are many such medications. Among the more commonly used ones are Pamelor, Tofranil, Prozac, Zoloft, Paxil, Effexor, Serzone, and Desyrel. Remeron, the newest on the market, has sedative side effects that may prove quite useful for bedtime use.

Stimulants

You have been aware, I bet, of the use of at least one stimulant to help in the management of headache pain for many years. Anacin and Empirin both combine caffeine with aspirin to produce a bigger pain-relieving bang for the buck. Caffeine in coffee or tea does help increase the effectiveness of analgesics, but for chronic pain patients stronger stimulants may well be more effective and appropriate. The most commonly used of these are Ritalin and

Dexedrine. Both come in immediate-release and sustained-release forms. Both not only counteract the sedative effects of narcotics but also enhance their pain-relieving abilities. The common side effects of disrupted sleep, nervousness, and reduced appetite can all be managed easily by starting with very low doses and confining routine usage to morning and afternoon.

Antihistamines and Neuroleptics

Many of these medications are chemically related. You have certainly heard of a few of them, such as Benadryl and Compazine. They can be used to help with nausea. Often they are used for the benefits of one of their side effects, such as to help with sleep. Benadryl is readily available without prescription. Less well known is the usefulness of these medications in pain management where they seem, in different ways from the stimulants, to improve responses to analgesics. In small amounts the neuroleptic Thorazine, originally developed as an anesthetic, has been used for decades to help in the management of severe chronic pain. Haldol is frequently used in hospices for help with severe pain. I find the new neuroleptic, Risperdal, in doses as low as one-quarter to one milligram to help many people significantly with essentially no side effects. For intractable pain, medications in this family should always be at least considered as useful helpers.

Muscle Relaxants and Other Special Medicines

The antianxiety agent Valium happens also to be an excellent muscle relaxant. Others that may be familiar to you are Flexeril and

Soma. A very excellent, powerful medication in this group, especially for pain originating from injured nerves, is Lioresal (baclofen). All muscle relaxants produce some sedation, but the sensitivity to this side effect varies widely from one individual to another. In a totally different category for help with chronic pain, if heart function is normal, is the drug called Mexitil (mexiletine). An oversimplified but approximate way of describing its effects is that it is like taking Novocain through your bloodstream, reducing the experience of pain.

Soporifics

Successful control over pain is not possible if a person suffers from significant sleep deprivation. Often reasonable sleep can be obtained if activity during the day is combined with appropriate relaxation techniques, certain herbal teas, appropriately aggressive use of analgesics, and, as needed, antianxiety agents. Sometimes, however, sleep medications, the soporifics, are needed. In this category, the safest totally nonaddicting compounds are Benadryl and Desyrel. (Desyrel, classified as an antidepressant, is actually a very effective sleep-inducing substance for many people.) The traditional sleeping pills used to include the barbiturates, especially Seconal. Most physicians no longer prescribe these highly addicting substances. Today's choices in the sleep-inducing department include Dalmane, Doral, Halcion, and Restoril. Dalmane often results in hangovers. Halcion can produce amnesia and confusion. Doral and Restoril have the same possible side effects; they just occur less frequently. Currently considered safer is Ambien, but it too is a central nervous system depressant that can create problems of memory and daytime drowsiness, particularly if used regularly. The now-popular hormone, melatonin, when used to help with sleep, has not been studied adequately. The currently available three-milligram doses may be from ten to one hundred times the amount necessary to supplement one's needs. No one knows the consequences of long-term use at this time, nor will we likely know for the next ten years.

The world of medications for pain and sleep is a very complex one. This is why you must be a participant in your pain treatment team, not accepting passively, without question, anything the doctor orders. Ask about side effects. Inquire about long-term effects and whether a medication can be taken every day. You are not challenging your doctors' training, experience, or authority when you seek to know all you can about what you are taking.

No matter how experienced or smart your doctors, only you know how you feel and how the various medications are affecting your body and mind. Even the smartest doctors are often in the dark when it comes to the very complex issues of drug-drug interactions. Have your own master list of prescribed medications and any other substances that you are taking. Also, you don't have to be a medical student to look things up in the two readily available books that describe medications, their uses, their side effects, and their known drug-drug interactions. These are the *Physicians' Desk Reference (PDR)* and the *Complete Drug Reference (CDR)*. The *PDR* simply reprints exactly the Food and Drug Administration required package inserts that describe, following government regulation, every approved drug. The print is small. There are more details than even most doctors care to read. I recommend the *CDR*, which is a publication of Consumer Reports Books in collaboration with the United States Pharmacopeia. This publication focuses much more on the needs of the consumer, emphasizing proper use of each medication and precautions to take while using the medication and listing side effects in an easier-to-follow fashion. Finally, I recommend that you order the U.S. Public Health Service's guides to the management of cancer pain through either the 1-800-4-CANCER telephone number or by writing for it at AHCPR Publications Clearinghouse, PO Box 8547, Silver Spring, MD 20907.

Appendix B: Nontraditional Treatment

THE OFFICE OF ALTERNATIVE MEDICINE of the National Institutes of Health, as noted in Chapter 5, defines five different nontraditional fields of practice: (1) alternative professionalized systems of health practice (traditional oriental medicine, Ayurvedic medicine, homeopathy, etc.); (2) adjunctive forms of health maintenance and healing (mind-body interventions, diet and nutrition, manual healing methods); (3) bioelectromagnetics; (4) pharmacologic and biologic treatments; (5) herbal medicine.

Alternative Professionalized Systems of Health Practice

While I list the various systems in order of the length of time they have been in use and by the attention they currently get, all actually are involved in the practice of healing and care in the United States.

Oriental Medicine

Unlike conventional Western medicine, having evolved from agrarian, tribal communities with shamanistic healers, all the oriental systems emphasize approaching the whole person in health and illness as that person's physical self and vital forces interact with nature: other living things, the sky, the earth, water. The views of life and philosophies of Taoism, Confucianism, and Buddhism have influenced the complex systems and techniques of oriental medicine as they have evolved over the last three thousand years. Each person is believed to have his or her own qi (chee), or spirit of life (the ancient Chinese had no concept of energy as such) that ebbs and flows throughout each day and throughout life. The relative balance and strength of this vital force accounts for wellness or ill health and connects one with all substances that have shape and form (rivers, sun, moon, earth, etc.). "Heaven and Earth contain Qi" (Wang Ch'ung, A.D. 27–100); that is, all things and people are made of qi. Qi has two opposing, always interacting realms, *yin* and *yang*. All natural phenomena are said to result from their interactions: *Yin* represents earth, woman, darkness, moon, absorbing forces; it presents itself through valleys and streams, broken lines, even numbers, the color orange; *yang* represents heaven, male, light, active, penetrating; it presents itself through mountains, the unbroken line, odd numbers, the color azure.

In ideal balance the flow of qi has a continuity with the vital forces of nature beyond the individual. The Chinese systems of health maintenance focus on keeping health and treating illness through various techniques designed to rebalance qi in the context of natural forces and facilitate its flow within and through the body's organ systems via channels whose directional landmarks are indicated by the acupuncture and acupressure points on the body. Our internal qi has phases and patterns of flow that are believed to repeat themselves twenty-five times each day and each night. Techniques of health maintenance and healing are believed to have spread with the Chinese culture and trade to Japan, Korea, Vietnam, and the Indian subcontinent.

In the United States a selection of systems has occurred based on those that appealed most in our culture. These are primarily acupuncture, massage, and herbal medicine. At this time only in New Mexico are oriental medical practices legally sanctioned with a scope of practice equivalent to that of primary-care medical and osteopathic physicians. The approach to the patient involves unhurried examination, particularly of the face, which is examined for skin color, temperature, and tension, for example; the patient is listened to; the patient's odors are noted; the patient is questioned about life habits, concerns, and symptoms; the patient's pulse is palpated for its characteristics.

Acupuncture was reviewed briefly in Chapter 5.

Acupressure uses the principles of acupuncture but without the use of needles. Fingertips or the hands of the therapist are used to stimulate selected acupoints, using varying degrees of pressure as well as applying pressure with different movements. This forms the basis of a number of systems of manual therapy increasingly known in the U.S. such as shiatsu and jin shin jyutsu. These systems of manual treatment are used for health maintenance as well as for treatment of specific health problems.

Moxibustion also uses acupuncture theories of practice and acupoints. Instead of needles or direct pressure, heat is applied to specific acupoints under the belief that intense, local heat helps the balance and flow of qi. Dried, crushed, and compacted leaves of dried *Artemesia vulgaris* (a perennial herb of the daisy family), sold in the form of cylinders or cones, are placed on tiny tinfoil/thick paper trays that are lit—much as one lights a stick of incense—and placed on the selected acupoints while the patient is lying down.

Moxibustion may be used by practitioners in combination with acupuncture and acupressure.

Cupping as used in oriental medicine also makes use of acupuncture theory of meridians, points, and channels for the flow of qi. In cupping, suction through the creation of a vacuum by warming small glass cups and overturning them on acupoints in areas suffering from congestion supposedly also rebalances qi, helping to disperse congestion as well as to help with sprains and arthritis. Interestingly, without regard to acupoints but with regard to congestion of the lungs and bronchitis, cupping has been used in Europe since at least the Middle Ages.

Remedial massage has formal written descriptions dating back to at least the second century B.C. Two major techniques are practiced. Ano uses a system of pressing and rubbing hand motions to enhance the well-being of the body. Tuina is a massage system that uses thrusting and rolling hand motions, also for the purpose of toning the body and improving the flow and balance of a person's qi.

Traditional Chinese medicine has a defined materia medica composed of 5,767 entries including herbs and more than three hundred extracts of minerals and animal products (*Encyclopedia of Traditional Chinese Medicine Substances*, 1977). Complex mixtures are directed toward toning and rebalancing the body, treating side effects, and directly treating the diseased organ or body function. Medications generally fall into categories based on the quality of their energy, classified as heating, cooling, drying, and moisturizing. Herbal medicine overlaps with ideas about nutrition that focus again on the energetic qualities of the food and the energetic need of the person in the context of activities and seasonal shifts. At best its use would be considered an adjunct to traditional cancer treatments.

Qi gong (pronounced "cheegung") refers to a system of healing more ancient than acupuncture. Qi gong integrates the use of breathing, meditation, and movement techniques to cleanse, strengthen, and improve the circulation of vital energy. As a healing system it is used to maintain health as well as to treat both acute and chronic conditions. Depending on the practitioner, it may or may not be combined with herbal medicine, utilizing ku qi, or the caloric energy from plants. Qi gong master healers use fa qi through "receiving" and "sending" hands to heal or improve ailments. (I have felt while in the same room with senior National Institutes of Health physicians fa qi by a qi gong master somehow transmitted over a distance of ten to fifteen feet and then observed as one of the scientists with severe posttennis tendinitis of the shoulder was "treated" without being touched, obtaining a significant reduction in pain within ten minutes—things we don't yet understand.)

How are the different oriental medicine techniques useful to cancer patients? *None of them cures cancer.* It is pure conjecture as to whether any of them through their effort to improve health helps in minimizing the risk of getting cancer or even preventing the development of some cancers. (The cancers have affected in different ways all people of all racial groups throughout time and continue to do so.) During treatment for cancer acupuncture, when performed properly, can help minimize or prevent chemotherapy-generated nausea. It also can often be helpful in moderating chronic pain.

All forms of oriental medicine as described here may be used alone or in combination to help cancer patients improve disrupted sleep and enhance diminished energy. They may facilitate the return to health and health maintenance once a person is in remission. There is little harm in these techniques. Objective data is limited about their usefulness, but one can assume a certain "consensual validation" because they have been used by tens of millions of people over at least two thousand years. All the oriental medicine techniques have the advantage of supportive, usually unpressured contact with a healer or sometimes in the context of a healing ceremony. The limiting factor in their use as complementary to your healing and recovery may be simply whether you believe in any particular technique and can pay for the services in which you choose to believe.

Ayurvedic Medicine

This ancient East Indian system of traditional Hindu medicine has in the last several years been highly touted as an extraordinary source of wisdom and healing. You will recognize in what follows that many of its basic tenets are no different from those of oriental medicine.

Its insights and some of its techniques and medicines are worthy of respect and further evaluation, but if it were anywhere as near to ultimate wisdom as some claim, I believe that Ayurvedic medicine would have been much more powerfully commanding in its influence centuries ago.

Ayus in Sanskrit means "life"; *veda* means "knowledge." The focus, unlike in oriental medicine, is on the conscious mind. Imbalancing forces or stresses on the mind are believed to lead to unhealthy lifestyles and unhealthy life decisions. These in turn promote ill health. Proper states of mind, often attained through the proper kinds of meditation, form the basic elements to Ayurvedic healing systems.

A patient (sufferer) is evaluated thoughtfully, including palpation of the pulse at the wrist. Toxins are removed through panchakarma: a combination of herbs to improve bowel function, herbal-based heat treatments, and herb-oil massages. Herbal medicines are prescribed based on the different evaluations of the patient. But these must be taken in conjunction with prescribed changes in diet, exercise (especially breathing and other yoga exercises), meditation exercises, and sleep. Goals include improved self-care through improved self-awareness and self-knowledge. Interpersonal and social health are supported, including methods directed toward proper diet as well as clean food and water. Ayurvedic medicine is state-supported in India. In the United States there is an American Association of Ayurvedic Medicine with a membership of between two and three hundred practitioners.

For Western cultures further objective evidence is needed to document where and how Ayurvedic medicine can be helpful.

Again, for believers it is undoubtedly helpful in maintaining hope and stabilizing health, particularly once a person is in remission. It offers at this time no exclusive, documented treatments for cancer. Some of its herbal preparations have been identified as having very interesting, biologically active effects and are being studied for both cancer prevention and anticancer properties. Some of these studies are supported by the National Institutes of Health. I recommend, as with oriental medicine, thoughtful caution and good common sense if you decide to adhere to Ayurvedic medicine as a form of treatment. Use it with but never instead of documented, well-known, and well-supervised forms of traditional treatment unless you have been informed by experienced oncologists that they have no further treatments to offer.

Homeopathic Medicine

Homeopathic medicine is both a philosophy of health and a formal system of drug therapeutics. Used widely in Europe, South America, and Asia, it was developed by German physician Samuel Hahnemann (1755–1843). During his lifetime many practices considered today essential elements of basic health care were either in their infancy or not yet known: sanitation, germ theory of disease/sterilization, immunization, anesthesia, antibiotics.

Hahnemann believed in the existence of a "vital force" in humans and other animals that could be mobilized and stabilized both to maintain health and to recover from disease. (*Homeo* derives from the Greek word for similar, *homoion*. *Pathy* derives from a Greek word *pathein* for disease or suffering.) Basic to Hahnemann's healing system of homeopathy is what he called the Law of Similars: "like shall be cured by like." His idea was that small doses of substances that can create symptoms, when given to a person suffering from that symptom—chills, fever, weakness, for example—encourage or kindle the person's vital force to rid itself of the symptom. He developed this idea while experimenting on himself with quinine bark in an effort to understand why it was an effective treatment for malaria, a disease whose initial symptoms are bouts of chills, fever, and weakness. This belief actually goes back in time to at least Hippocrates (460–377 B.C.). Hahnemann further elaborated on this belief by proposing that "small drug doses kindle vital forces; moderate doses can increase them; large dose depress them, the largest doses remove them." One example is the plant substance *Nux vomica*, also known as poison nut/Quacker Button or simply the seeds of an evergreen plant; it contains chemicals known as alkaloids that can be powerful toxins—strychnine is one—but that are used in extremely diluted forms to treat gastrointestinal disorders. Gastrointestinal symptoms are among the first signs of poisoning by strychnine and other alkaloids.

Some of Hahnemann's other principles of practice include the Doctrine of Signatures, Potentization, and Indispositions. The Doctrine of Signatures says that a plant intended for medicinal use has within it a sign or signature in the form of color, smell, or other characteristic that indicates its use in healing. Potentization refers to the basic system in homeopathy of repeatedly diluting with water/alcohol solutions and shaking medicines (which may derive from animal, vegetable, or mineral sources) to the appropriate point—"the higher the potency of a homeopathic preparation, the smaller the amount of substance present in solution"—for the condition that is being treated. Indispositions refers to Hahnemann's belief that many illnesses are brought on by errors in habits of living, environmental factors, or work worries. (This concept, also basic to oriental and Ayurvedic medicine, is rearticulated by many others based on studies from environmental medicine/public health and psychiatry/psychology. It has taken firm hold of health policy and law over the last twenty years with regard to pollution control, "sick building" laws, tobacco and alcohol control, and industrial and personal stress management programs.)

Homeopathy as a system claims to be helpful with health promotion as well as the treatment of acute and chronic health conditions. It assumes that all disease states reflect themselves in the patient's consciousness in the form of altered moods and thinking, changes in sensation, and perceptible alterations in the function and appearance of parts of the body. It claims that adherence to its principles will increase one's resistance to disease, heighten one's sense of well-being, and quicken recovery from acute illness. A 1993 study estimated that 1 percent of the U.S. population sought help from homeopathic doctors.

In actual practice properly trained and certified homeopathic physicians spend a great deal of time—up to two hours in their initial consultations—with patients. Tending to use fewer drugs and order fewer lab tests than conventional physicians, they exhort the patient to realize that treatments often take a long time to act, working against the impatience of our "quick fix" culture. Costs of homeopathy over time are therefore often lower. Homeopathic remedies are regulated in their manufacture by the U.S. Food and Drug Administration, but their effectiveness is not subject to scientific review and substantiation. Much more research is needed to objectively determine the effectiveness of homeopathic remedies in acute and chronic conditions.

Obviously the homeopathic health system believes it can contribute to cancer prevention. It does contribute in terms of calling for adherence to its doctrine of Indispositions. However, once a person has cancer, homeopathy offers "constitutional treatments" in addition to the traditional medical treatments of surgery, chemotherapy, and radiation. Homeopathic physicians do accept the usefulness of conventional medical treatments for the cancers.

Homeopaths believe that they can improve the quality of life of cancer patients during active treatment and especially during remission. If you choose to seek care from a homeopath, he or she may or may not be a licensed physician. Only Arizona, Connecticut, and Nevada currently have licensing boards for homeopathic physicians. A homeopath should present certification diplomas from either the National Center for Homeopathy (Alexandria, Virginia) or the American Institute of Homeopathy (made up of medical and osteopathic physicians), which gives professional certification through its American Board of Homeotherapeutics, yielding a *D. Ht.* after the professional's name.

Naturopathic Medicine

Licensed naturopathic doctors (N.D.s) are found in seven states and Canada. They are trained at three different schools, one in Washington State, one in Oregon, and one in Arizona. Originating as a field of practice in the United States, it integrates herbal (botanical) medicine, nutrition, massage, manipulative techniques, and hydrotherapy. The focus of N.D.s is on the body's natural healing capacities, the doctor's role as a teacher, disease prevention through a healthy lifestyle, and treatment of the whole person. Some of the herbs used may be helpful with specific disease states such as irritable bowel, hypertension, and even viral infections. Naturopaths may spend significant amounts of time with their patients. Their craft offers no special treatments for cancer but may offer some help in regaining health after active treatment for cancer.

Environmental Medicine

This form of medicine emphasizes what its name suggests: that the environment and its many elements influence the genetic predispositions of individuals. Hence much time is spent on determining allergies and other sensitivities and subsequently on educating the patient. Many laboratory tests are taken. Avoidance of particular food antigens may be urged aggressively as may be encouragement to alter one's environment so as to avoid toxins such as formaldehyde fumes from compressed fiber board. This system makes claims in terms of cancer prevention but none in terms of cancer treatment.

Anthroposophically Extended Medicine

Another system whose name refers to wisdom: *sophia*, the root for wisdom; *anthropos*, the root for human. Developed by an Austrian scientist and philosopher in the late nineteenth to early twentieth century, this system took form in collaboration with a Dutch physician named Ita Wegman. Training as a medical doctor is considered essential. Anthroposophically extended medicine integrates such traditional training with elements of homeopathy and naturopathy. It thus uses "potentized" medications and herbal medications. It also emphasizes an integration of the spiritual and physical self. How the rhythms of life influence the effectiveness of medications and the responses of people to medications is studied and utilized. This system too claims the capacity to improve the health of individuals. It also has been a focal point for studies of the anticancer properties of the plant mistletoe and its metabolites.

Adjunctive Forms of Health Maintenance and Healing

Mind-Body Interventions

These interventions are today often associated with the writings and teachings of a Harvard professor of medicine Herbert Benson (*The Relaxation Response*), the former *Saturday Review* editor turned UCLA Medical School faculty member Norman Cousins (*Anatomy of an Illness as Perceived by the Patient*), the MacArthur scholar and director of Commonweal Michael Lerner (*Choice in Healing*), and the former New Haven–based and Yale-affiliated surgeon Bernie Siegel (*Love, Medicine, and Miracles*). In truth mind-body interventions encompass a philosophy that is thousands of years old about the mind/body/spirit/environment that is encompassed in both oriental and Ayurvedic medicine. Specific mind-body therapies include some discussed elsewhere in this book and some not previously listed. My list includes the different forms of individual and group psychotherapy; the different forms and schools of meditation training (Zen, yoga, TM, healing prayer, etc.); the relaxation response (through breathing, focusing, and biofeedback techniques); guided imagery; hypnosis/self-hypnosis; yoga; dance therapy; music therapy; art therapy.

All these techniques involve expressing oneself in particular ways, quieting oneself down from a hypervigilant state, focusing one's mind/thoughts/feelings, and communicating with one's body. All clearly help different individuals deal with cancer-induced loss of control, uncertainty, and helplessness. Therefore they can unquestionably help with quality of life. Excellent traditional research has documented this, particularly with respect to professionally led group therapy. Group therapy for cancer patients enhances the quality of life for most participants and for some seems to prolong life expectancy, according to several well-designed prospective studies. The mechanisms for these positive effects are currently unknown. I find myself recommending to cancer patients participation in a group for the first year postdiagnosis.

Diet and Nutrition

Both diet and nutrition are clearly important in the maintenance of health, the prevention of various disease states, and the promotion of healing. The problems of the modern "affluent" diet are now widely known, as are the nutritional guidelines presented by the National Academy of Sciences and presented through the U. S. Department of Agriculture's food pyramid (1990). Astoundingly, most major U.S. hospital centers still do not fully comply with these nutritional guidelines. Active longitudinal research into the role of vitamin and mineral supplements in health maintenance and healing in chronic diseases is under way. All supplemental vitamins and minerals can be toxic over time when ingested in high doses—more is not necessarily safe, much less better!

Orthomolecular medicine involves the use of high-dose nutrient therapy for illnesses ranging from cancers to schizophrenia. The focus has often been on certain vitamins like vitamin C or B_3. Some interesting data exists about the usefulness of vitamin C as well as a substance called coenzyme Q_{10}. However, at this time there is no scientific support for the exclusive usefulness of high-dose nutrient therapy in any specific health condition despite many active, aggressive claims to the contrary.

Macrobiotic diets for cancer are based on the belief that diet is among the factors that allow the development of cancer. Believing that overconsumption of milk, cheese, meats, eggs, iced drinks, and soft drinks produces toxins, macrobiotics dips into the oriental theory of yin and yang forces, attributing yin or yang values to different foods. Macrobiotic diets minimize the consumption of animal products and emphasize the use of whole grain cereals, beans, lentils, and vegetables and specific styles of cooking food. These are then prescribed based on the kind of cancer a patient has and its relationship to such opposing forces, the goal being, as always, a re-balancing of the patient's system.

There are at least two other cancer diet systems: the Livingston/Wheeler system and the Wigmore treatment. The former diet claims to enhance the body's antitumor capacity. The latter relies on a defined fruit/vegetable/grain combination that supposedly enhances health. While no quality longitudinal studies support the effectiveness of any of these diets, no known harm is associated with any of them as long as the person is making himself or herself also available to treatments of known effectiveness. For many, adhering to a specific diet becomes a focal point for family and friendship support, a predictable area where one has some reality of control. Hence participation for some is both comforting and a form of proactive expression of autonomy.

Vegetarian diets come in many forms. The most extreme form is the vegan diet, which allows for no animal products or products derivative of animals. Medically, a very interesting variation on the theme is the lacto-ovo-vegetarian diet of the Seventh Day Adventists—they eat no red meat, fish, or poultry. The overall cancer death rate for adherent males is about half that of the U.S. population and for females about 70 percent that of the general population. These statistical associations are particularly strong with respect to cancers of the colon and rectum. This does make you wonder!

Manual Healing Methods

These methods are discussed in Chapter 5.

Osteopathic Medicine

Sometimes what was definitely alternative, nonestablishment medicine becomes very much part of the mainstream. Osteopathic medicine is the best example of such a change. There are more than thirty-two thousand osteopathic physicians in the United States alone. They are licensed to practice medicine and surgery in all fifty states, equal to medical doctors. This is quite an accomplishment for a philosophy of learning and treating started in the late nineteenth century by a medical school dropout who originally promoted himself for rapid bonesetting and "magnetic" healing. Osteopathic medicine emphasizes the observation that form and function in the human body are interdependent phenomena. Diseases are considered to be based on disruptions of normal anatomic, physiologic, and behavioral interactions. Eight basic manipulative techniques are used to improve function. Many of these techniques are found in other forms of manipulative therapies. Today's osteopaths use manipulative techniques in combination with traditional medical diagnostics and therapeutics. They are generally excellent primary-care doctors; indeed, at least 60 percent of them have chosen to focus on primary-care treatment.

Chiropractic

This method of treatment also originated in the late nineteenth century. The founder was a grocer who had an intense interest in and a gift for healing: D. D. Palmer. Over the years he and his sons developed a system of treatment based on his theory that joint dysfunction and joint misalignment are responsible for many forms of illness. Today more than forty-five thousand practitioners exist in the United States, treating as much as 12 percent of the population. Chiropractors may not prescribe drugs or perform surgery. They manipulate joints and soft tissues using thrusting as well as high-velocity techniques. They make no claims about curing or treating the cancers.

Massage Therapies

Massage therapies are described in Chapter 5.

Biofield Therapeutics

This is the generic term for what is popularly called the "laying on of hands" or "therapeutic touch." With many of these techniques the patient experiences the hands of the healer near his or her body but rarely actually touching as in the massage therapies. These therapeutics are found in the most ancient of healing ceremonies in many cultures of the world. Besides the preceding terms you may have heard of energy healing, qi gong, Reiki, and Shen therapy. Proponents include practitioners and patients. They find that these therapeutic techniques decrease an individual's feelings of stress, decrease feelings of depression, and improve function.

Craniosacral Therapy

This technique represents a gentle hands-on approach to improving the alignment and flow of physiologic processes, particularly among the bones of the skull (including facial and jaw bones), entire spine (including sacrum and coccyx), and pelvis. Noninvasive, its purpose is to normalize abnormal tensions and reduce stresses on the meningeal membranes (the coverings of the brain and spinal cord). An osteopathic physician, John Upledger, is the major advocate of this therapy. Besides being comforting to patients, it supposedly improves the functioning of the immune system, the central nervous system, the endocrine system, and the visceral organs.

Physical Therapy

Developed during World War I to aid the rehabilitation and healing of the wounded, physical therapy combines elements of many of the preceding manual therapies with the use of heat and cold, ultrasound, electrical stimulation, traction, splinting and other physical supports, ambulatory training, therapeutic stretching, therapeutic exercises, and a great deal of patient education as part of the entire process of care. Its focus is improved physical function: improved posture, flexibility, strength, endurance, and mobility. Referred to as *physiotherapy* in Europe, its practitioners in the United States all receive formal, degree training based on courses of study, supervision, and examinations; all are licensed.

Of the 120,000 or so practitioners today, many unfortunately are depending more and more on the more lucrative use of mechanical and electrical devices as well as hot and cold packs rather than the more labor-intensive and tiring educational and manual techniques. The best physical therapists combine all the approaches available to them in a manner tailored to the needs of each patient. When this is done, their work is significantly complementary to that of physicians and nurses on behalf of all individuals with chronic health problems and cancer in particular. Their work is reimbursed by health insurance.

Bioelectromagnetics

Bioelectromagnetics refers to the fascinating field in medicine that studies the electromagnetic systems of living bodies and through those studies develops methods for enhancing healing and health and treating conditions such as pain. You have doubtless heard of at least two applications of this area of medical science: pulsed electromagnetic field devices that assist significantly in bone healing, particularly in areas where blood circulation is less than optimal; and nerve and spinal cord stimulation to help with the control of chronic pain. What follows is a brief discussion of two additional areas of specific interest in treating cancer using different forms of bioelectromagnetics.

Immune System Stimulation

Research in this area indicates that electromagnetic stimulation may be a double-edged sword. Chronic, long-term exposure such as can occur when living next to high-tension power lines may suppress immune system functioning. (Very recent studies show no support for this concern.) On the other hand, short-term exposure may possibly augment the activity of natural killer cells, which are very important members of the cancer-fighting team. Studies continue. Caution is warranted at this time.

Neuroendocrine Modulations

Melatonin, a pituitary hormone, is believed to help in stopping the growth of cancer cells as well as in regulating our day-night biologic rhythms. Its secretion can be stimulated by some electromagnetic fields and suppressed by others. Stimulation by electromagnetic fields could be useful in cancer treatment if we could figure out what precise magnetic field characteristics and strengths work.

Alternative Pharmacological and Biological Treatments

Alternative pharmacologic and biologic treatments include biologic treatments that have developed a dedicated following at different times during this century without acceptance by mainstream medicine because of the absence of well-designed experiments evaluating their toxicity and effectiveness. Advocates for these many different substances have always claimed that they are nontoxic but have not provided convincing objective evidence to support such claims.

As a group these treatments are comprised of both drugs and vaccines. All are subject to controversy. Most seem to be directed toward improving the functioning of the immune system. All actually raise intriguing research questions about different approaches to improving the treatment of cancer. Some are specific substances such as the antineoplastons (fragments, called *peptides*, of proteins from urine and blood), shark and other forms of animal cartilage, 714-X, MTH-68, and Iscador/mistletoe. They all in some form may eventually be found to have anticancer activity, but many substances—such as plain old bleach—do. The unanswered questions about these substances or combinations of substances are how active their anticancer cell activity is, how long it lasts, and *at what cost to the healthy cells and structures in the person.* Others, such as immuno-augmentative therapy, the Hoxsey method, Essiac, and Rivici's guided chemotherapy, are systems of treatment using combinations of substances that are intended both to kill cancer cells and to promote the body's antitumor activity. Although considered very eccentric by mainstream medicine, they too may present useful ideas for possible investigation of biologic functions relevant to the war on cancer.

Herbal Medicine

"I know cancer of the breast is often thought to be incurable, yet we have here in town a kind of shell made of some wood . . . which has done wonders in this disease."

Benjamin Franklin, in a letter to his sister, 1731

Herbal medicines (phytomedicines) are found in all cultures of the world. These are the plant-derived medications discovered by trial and error, then incorporated into folklore and native healing arts. Many of today's most basic medicines have such origins: digitalis, aspirin, curare, the ergot medications, vincristine, Taxol, and many more. Herbal medicines in their natural form are poorly regulated for quality and safety in the United States. We still, for example, allow the sale of comfrey root, a highly toxic herbal remedy taken off the market by Canada and other countries. Herbal medicines are a growing industry, now reaching $1.5 billion in annual U.S. sales. Deadly pennyroyal oil, cohosh, ephedra, and many others are easily available. The FDA MEDWATCH program may be of assistance to you if you are thinking about any herbal medicine. You can reach it by calling 1-800-FDA-1088 or you can fax for information at 1-800-FDA-0178.

Phytomedicines that may prove to have some relevance to cancer patients follow.

Milk thistle (*Silybum marianum*) may protect from certain forms of radiation damage. Intravenous extracts are used in the emergency rooms of some European countries as part of treating liver poisoning from toxic chemicals.

Ginkgo biloba, an herb of Asian origin, is widely used in Europe to stimulate circulation including in the retina, lower cholesterol, and modify hypertension. It possibly could be helpful in recovery postsurgery and after radiation for brain tumors.

Echinacea (purple cornflower) has been written about extensively. Data suggests that it provides nonspecific stimulation of the immune system. It may help to fight bacterial infections. It also seems to increase lymphocyte secretion of tumor necrosis factor as well as interleukin 1 and 6.

Baical skullcaproot, coptis rhizome, woad leaf, wild chrysanthemum flower, and purple-skinned garlic bulbs are among the Chinese phytomedicines that have antibacterial and antiviral activity. Some experiments show that they work together with modern antibiotics, yielding better clinical results—that is, the patients get better faster.

Cancer and Nontraditional Treatments

An examination of alternative medicine reminds us that mankind has struggled for centuries to improve health and reduce suffering. A time line just from the eighteenth century reveals an almost unbroken series of remedies proposed and promoted to cure cancer. Some have been herbal; some have been mineral; some have been chemical; some a mixture of all three. Others have included various forms of "cosmic energy treatment," light, and sound therapies. Behind these treatments and their creators lie various intellectual, personal, and social factors. They are sustained by the desire to maintain hope, to trust, to be cared for, to be "made better." Those deserving of our trust will allow themselves to be examined through the Western scientific method, a severe system of systematic information gathering and observations whose purpose is to measure, describe, and differentiate between wishes or promises and real change at the molecular, cellular, organ-system, or whole-person level. Its only profit is its intellectual honesty, its integrity, and its potential to protect us all from our wishes of magic.

Appendix C: Special Community Resources

SURPRISING AS IT IS to many people, helpful resources beyond immediate family and friends do exist in the community for all people with serious chronic illnesses. If you need assistance or information, don't be shy: inquire. The richness of what is available if you reach out to discover what is there can make a very important difference to you. Local branches of your cancer advocacy organization always offer help, as do community service organizations; religious congregations; community hospitals; county health, rehabilitation, and social service offices; and libraries. I present the following only to give you some ideas, to get you started in obtaining for yourself and your family as much support as you can reasonably attain.

Assistance with the Cost of Medication

Prescription Drug Indigent Program of the Pharmaceutical Manufacturers Association:

PMA
1100 Fifteenth St., N.W.
Washington, DC 20005
1-800-PMA-INFO or (202) 393-5200

Many of the major pharmaceutical firms and some of the smaller ones provide medications at either significantly reduced costs or without cost for people with special needs. Letters of medical necessity as well as supporting financial documents are needed.

Transportation

Corporate Angel Network (CAN): transportation on corporate aircraft at no cost on a space-available basis to treatment centers and to home can be obtained; the patient must be able to walk onto the aircraft; preapproval and medical authorization are needed.

CAN
Westchester County Airport, Building 1
White Plains, NY 10604
(914) 328-1313

Wings of Freedom helps find discounted commercial airline tickets for patients and their family members for travel to treatment centers and their homes.

Wings of Freedom
Box 160
Rural Hall, NC 27045
(919) 969-9122

National Patient Air Transportation Assistance Hotline: assistance with transportation problems and tickets.

1-800-296-1217

Income

Social Security and Supplemental Social Security Income: these federally funded programs may be able to provide assistance; call for information on eligibility:

1-800-SSA-1213

The Internal Revenue Service, believe it or not, not only will provide helpful information concerning necessary nonmedical expenses for which you can claim deductions, including travel but also will help in deferral of tax filings and tax payments based on special needs, as well as income averaging. The key to getting help is to ask in advance.

Social Assistance

Local foundations, charities, and local service organizations often give small (less than $1,000) cash grants to provide emergency assistance for nonmedical expenses such as with utilities, equipment rental, and transportation.

Homemakers, home health aides, and companion services can be obtained through a variety of sources. Contacting your nearest local chapter of the American Cancer Society is often a good place to start. Its location and telephone number can be obtained through a central directory:

1-800-ACS-2345

If you have a Visiting Nurses Association in your area, it too can often be of assistance. Finally, many local benevolent associations, business clubs, churches, synagogues, mosques, and temples have trained volunteers who assist, particularly with transportation and companionship.

Work

Know your rights, particularly under both the Federal Rehabilitation Act of 1973 and the 1992 revision of the Americans with Disabilities Act. I suggest everyone read the National Coalition for Cancer Survivorship booklet entitled *Working It Out: Your Employment Rights*. Call (301) 650-8868 to order a copy.

Your county and state Bureau of Vocational Rehabilitation can often provide guidance concerning local laws protecting you as well as available retraining programs if needed.

Legal Assistance

Again, consult your local American Cancer Society. In addition, obtain information that might be relevant from:

National Coalition for Cancer Survivorship
(301) 650-8868

American Association for Retired Persons
Health Advocacy Services Office
601 E St., N.W.
Washington, DC 20049

Of concern most frequently is information about living wills and powers of attorney.

Hospice

Even small, relatively rural communities often have home hospice services. If you need these services, you also need to know whether they meet basic state liscensing requirements as to the composition, supervision, and quality of their staff. For general information and guidelines, write to:

National Hospice Organization
1901 N. Moore St., Suite 901
Arlington, VA 22209

Appendix D: The Future

IN SEPTEMBER 1995 the U.S. Food and Drug Administration proposed new regulations to allow for more rapid introduction of experimental treatments. Supported by the president, these regulations were signed into law in 1996. This section gives you one brief overview of some of the extraordinary approaches to treatment that are in the process of being studied or used. Many of them derive from similar technologies or are used in combination with more standard treatments. We will look at the new technologies, surgery and organ transplantation, radiation therapies, chemotherapies, infection control, fatigue control, bone marrow and stem cell transplants, the immunotherapies, and finally genetics and gene therapy. After that, we will discuss some of the exciting developments in early identification and prevention.

New Technologies

We continue to find new technologies applied to all areas of cancer care—prevention; early diagnosis; surgical, radiotherapy, and chemotherapy treatments. They also form the basis of many innovative treatments. In Chapter 11, we reviewed some of these technologies, such as chemotherapy infusion pumps, indwelling catheters, and fiber-optics (a technology that renders diagnostic and surgical procedures less invasive and less traumatic). Others involve more sophisticated uses of familiar home items such as the telephone and television.

For example, the exploding technology of high-definition, digitalized transmission of auditory and visual information over fiber-optic telephone lines or from communication satellites constitutes the basis for the rapid evolution of telemedicine. Telemedicine is already used in some hospitals as a method for bringing expertise not locally available into operating rooms at the time of surgery. Expert consultation can also be obtained in this fashion on x-rays, CAT scans, MRIs, and tissues pathology.

When the cold war ended, specialized military technologies in development became available for civilian use, fostering improvements in existing diagnostic systems. One example involves refinements of ultrasound imaging so that high-definition imaging (HDI) is now possible. HDI systems in the proper hands can distinguish between noncancerous and cancerous breast lumps. The development of three-dimensional rotating delivery excitation off resonance MRI systems (3-D RODEO MRI) is another example. These not yet widely available systems give image clarity that is twenty times higher than existing MRIs, with better contrast of visualized tissues. They actually allow visualization of how much a cancerous breast mass extends into surrounding tissue. When available to everyone, this technology will permit breast-conserving surgery combined with radiation treatments to become more of an option.

Another approach uses improved radioactive tracers combined with traditional diagnostic techniques such as x-ray mammography as a way to obtain more accurate characterization of breast lumps. For other forms of cancer a technique called *PET scanning (positron-emission tomography)*, which because of its expense has been used primarily for research, in combination with radioactive tracers sensitive to lung tissue, may allow earlier diagnosis of lung cancer sometime in the future as well as the accurate determination of whether or not it has spread beyond the lungs.

Photodynamic therapy (PDT) represents another innovative approach to treatment. It relies on expertise from organic chemistry and physics. Today two families of special light-sensitive chemical compounds are being evaluated for cancer treatment. One family is related to the chemicals in our red blood cells that carry oxygen, the hematoporphyrins. Specially engineered forms of these chemicals, when exposed to light (laser source), produce energized oxygen (singlet oxygen); oxygen in this form is highly destructive (toxic) to all cells with which it comes in contact.

These chemicals are harmless without light stimulation. One form, approved for use in Canada, called Photofrin II, helps fight recurrent, localized bladder cancer. The patient needs to avoid sunlight for two months after treatment with this compound—the length of time it takes the body to excrete Photofrin. A newer member of this family, BDT (benzo-porphyrin), apparently can be excreted within twenty-four hours. The other family of compounds derives from a Nile River weed. They are called *psoralens* and are activated by ultraviolet light. They enter cells easily. When such cells are exposed to ultraviolet light, the psoralens make the cell DNA strands stick together, preventing the cell from dividing.

PDT has been known since the 1970s. To this point its cancer-fighting abilities have failed to produce dramatic results; however, as an adjunctive therapy, especially for those cancers near the surface of the bladder, on the peritoneal lining, or cutaneous chest wall breast cancer recurrences PDT may prove to be increasingly useful in the future.

Surgery and Organ Transplantation

Organ transplantation—kidney, liver, pancreas, heart, lungs—is continuing to develop as a special surgical field. In cancer treatment, liver transplantation can now allow for good survival when combined with complete removal of tumor-filled livers in children. Over the coming years undoubtedly organ transplantation will become an important element of successful treatment for selected cancers, just as bone marrow transplantation has assumed a more important role in cancer therapy.

In the past, amputations were at times considered the only surgical treatment possible. For some years now amputations are performed much less frequently. They have been replaced successfully with various forms of limb-sparing surgeries in which cancerous bone and tissue is removed and then replaced with metal and plastic grafts. Also, new techniques of grafting have evolved such as microvascular free tissue transfer, thanks to the development of surgeries performed under microscopes. This allows the successful reconnection of tiny blood vessels and nerves. These techniques as well as improved technologies for implants, biocomposite grafts (using, for example, radiation-sterilized donor bone), and prosthetics all allow significantly better cosmetic and functional results in cancer surgery, especially of the head, neck, and face, than was dreamed of twenty years ago. The quality of healing and the quality of life for patients have been enhanced significantly.

Intraoperative ultrasound images help guide special probes through which liquid nitrogen can flow into cancer masses, freezing the cancer cells to death. This is called *cryosurgery*. Certain deep tumors such as in the liver can be treated this way, avoiding cutting into and through healthy tissue, producing fewer complications, and allowing shorter hospital stays.

Another example involves the use of lasers. Carbon dioxide lasers allow for successful treatment, with little trauma to the patient, of cancerous changes on the cervix. Much more aggressive removal of tumor masses within the peritoneal cavity can also be accomplished more safely with laser surgery than with other techniques. And, for a final example, computer-assisted volumetric stereotaxic surgery (COMPASS) proves a very useful technique for reducing the risk of injury to normal brain tissue. As a result, it reduces operating room and hospital time, improves outcomes, and allows for surgical destruction of tumors deep in the brain.

New Approaches in Radiation Therapies

Several new ways of applying radiation therapy (also called *radiotherapy*) are being developed today. In interstitial therapy or brachytherapy seeds of short-lived radioactive material are actually placed, using special visualization techniques, directly into tumor masses. In the future this technique may replace much of the surgery currently performed on prostate cancers localized to that gland. Gamma knife radiotherapy uses three-dimensional targeting to focus gamma radiation from multiple cobalt-60 sources on precise cancerous tissue targets. In intraoperative radiotherapy higher doses can be delivered directly to areas with cancer that have been exposed by surgery without directly radiating other tissues. Proton radiotherapy, available in only a few major treatment centers, is for tumors located in very-difficult-to-reach places. Finally, radioactive materials attached to monoclonal antibodies are being produced in laboratories to attach to specific types of cancer cells (true "magic bullets").

Radiation treatments have effects that are immediate, called *acute* (hours to weeks); intermediate, called *subacute* (weeks to months); and *long term* (more than six months). Skin redness, irritation of the mucous membrane linings of the body, and alterations in bowel and bladder function and fertility are some of the acute affects. These involve the normal, rapidly dividing cells of the body and are similar to chemotherapy side effects. Subacute effects include the preceding as well as possible changes in salivary gland function and inflammation of the lungs, heart, and kidneys. Long-term effects can be most disturbing, involving the liver and the brain. They range from increased risk of new cancer (meningiomas, gliomas of the nerve tissue, sarcomas, leukemias) to sterility, damage to pituitary function, and reduction of cognitive function.

Collaboration with other medical specialists allows for accurate identification of individuals who are unusually sensitive or vulnerable to radiation so that proper protective measures can be taken before treatments. Such collaborations also allow improved, innovative multimodal treatments such as the use of high-dose cisplatin and radiotherapy for advanced disease, or radiotherapy used with biologic modifiers such as cytokines or monoclonal antibodies. All these improvements are terribly important since almost 60 percent of cancer patients in the United States will have some radiation therapy during the course of their illness.

Improvements in radiotherapy continue every year. Tissues around radiation sites that are difficult to protect can now be shielded as a result of collaborations between polymer chemists and metallurgists. This yields substances called *elastomeric polymers* that can be molded to fit different contours and shapes in difficult places such as the head, mouth, neck, and groin. Layers of these polymers can be filled with heavy metal powders such as copper, tin, and zinc that will diffuse radiation beams. When this is combined with three-dimensional simulation as part of treatment planning, greater sparing of critical structures results. In the process of development and use are chemicals such as amifostine (Ethyol) that when given to patients before radiation therapy enhance the ability of normal tissues to resist damage from radiation treatments.

Radiation does decrease healing, the proliferation of normal cells, and the return of blood vessels to bring oxygen to and nourish newly growing healthy tissues. This may result in fluid retention (edema), poor wound healing with ulceration and infection, and even the death of underlying bone (bone necrosis). Even exposure to 100 percent oxygen has been shown to be insufficient to give enough oxygen to irradiated tissues for proper wound healing. Recent work using hyperbaric oxygen chambers with head and neck cancer patients after radiation, but before reconstruction of disfigured sites, has yielded repair success rates of up to 93 percent! These results seem well worth the considerable effort—thirty ninety-minute hyperbaric sessions at 2.4 times normal atmospheric pressure before reconstructive surgery and ten such sessions post-surgery. Future improvements building on these successes generate much hope.

New Approaches in Chemotherapy

Because of the incredibly rapid development of our understanding of the structures and functioning of cells, chemotherapeutic agent development no longer is as primitive as simply searching for new cell poisons. Agents currently used plus those in development are now selected based on understanding of how they influence cell structure (cell membrance, cell organelles, cell nucleus) and function (particularly the cell manufacture of the proteins and enzymes that allow cell division, cell longevity, and the self-destruction of aged, defective, or unneeded cells, also called *apoptosis*). Thus the search for improved chemotherapies focuses on discovering new compounds that are even more effective in arresting the growth of or killing cancer cells. Many different mechanisms are being studied. These include inhibiting cytoplasmic metabolism, disrupting the function of cytoplasmic organelles, disrupting the cell's ability to replicate, attacking cancer-causing genes (oncogenes and protooncogenes and their protein products), and disrupting the environment of cancer cells by blocking the development of new blood vessels (angiogenesis).

Interesting new compounds in development include synthetic retinoids such as polyprenoic acid for the treatment of liver cancer;

the P-30 protein (Onconas) derived from the skin of the leopard frog for cancer of the linings of the lungs, chest, and abdomen (mesotheliomas); irinotecan (Camptosar) for metastic colorectal cancer; Hycamtin for ovarian cancer; and flutamide (Eulexin) for advanced prostate cancer.

Much effort today is therefore directed toward several other dimensions of treatment. These include (1) knowing what are the best combinations of agents (combined therapy) to use for different cancers; (2) determining before treatment, especially in relapsed cancers, the sensitivity of the specific cancer as determined in cell culture sensitivity tests (predictive anticancer drug sensitivity tests) to different chemotherapeutic agents and combinations of agents; (3) minimizing or preventing cancer cells from becoming unresponsive to different chemical agents after a time (acquired multidrug resistance); (4) determining not only how much medication to give on the basis of body size but also what quantity is best given in a rapid amount of time (bolus) or over a prolonged period of time (constant infusion) to optimize the tumor-killing effect—possibly including very-high-dose treatments combined with "rescue" of the patient's immune and hematologic systems through stem cell support; (5) determining the best time during the course of the treatment process and even during the day-night cycle (circadian timing) for administration of a particular chemotherapeutic agent (our immune system activity and hormone levels vary greatly over a twenty-four-hour period, and this influences both response to chemotherapeutic agents and the toxicity we suffer).

When surgery or radiation is considered the primary treatment for a particular cancer, the use of chemotherapy following such treatment is called *adjuvant chemotherapy*. Its purpose is to improve the outcome by decreasing the incidence of recurring local, regional, or distant metastases. Clinical research continuously evaluates what combinations, in what doses (high or low), delivered over how much time, produce the best disease-free outcomes. Examples include the different uses of the platinum-based compounds (cisplatin and carboplatin) in combination with standard chemotherapy agents such as doxorubicin, 5-fluorouracil, or cyclophosphamide. Collaborative multi-institutional studies attempt to decipher when chemotherapy is best used as adjuvant treatment and when it is best used as the primary treatment. For instance, women whose breast cancer stage and age seem, in combination, to put them at substantial risk for systemic metastases do better when given twelve weeks of chemotherapy, followed by radiation therapy, rather than radiation treatment first after lumpectomy.

You have undoubtedly heard of the antiestrogen hormone tamoxifen (Nolvadex) as well as the progesterone-blocking hormone called RU-486. Both inhibit cancer cell growth. Other hormones such as the corticosteroids (prednisone, dexamethasone, etc.) down-regulate the inflammatory response. In combination with chemotherapy, corticosteroids often can give improved pain control. Some synthetic hormonelike compounds modify the action of naturally occurring steroids but also are directly toxic to cancer cells. A well-known example of such a compound used to help cancer patients is called Megace. Medications that alter hormone flow from the pituitary gland are made of protein fragments (peptides). These peptides block gonadotropin secretion. As a result, steroid production in ovaries and testes and adrenals is suppressed. One example is called Lupron, used widely in metastatic prostate cancer treatment.

Infection and Pain Control: Future Directions

Biofilms are essentially slime within which large clumps of bacteria successfully hide, the slime being composed of overlapping fibers of complex sugar molecules (polysaccharides). Biofilms coat many surfaces that seem clean in the home and in the hospital, exposing an immunosuppressed cancer patient to danger. Understanding this reality generates new techniques for improved sanitation of surfaces, instruments, catheters, and the human mouth.

You will note the constant development of new antifungal and antibiotic medicines. Since many cancer patients used to die of infections, these new medicines are critical. These medications may, however, complicate the treatment process and your quality of life because some, such as the quinolone antibiotics (e.g., Cipro), can produce significant side effects such as insomnia, depression, confusion, difficulty walking, and even agitation to the point of psychosis. (So don't blame your cancer or chemotherapy for something weird when it may be something as ordinary as an antibiotic that you are taking.)

A natural chemical called *prostaglandin* can now be synthesized (called misoprostol), which when used as a mouth rinse decreases (if used before treatment) the mouth ulcers that may develop from radiation therapy. New anesthetics and new anesthetic creams continue to be introduced. One of these, a cream (oil in water emulsion) combining lidocaine and prilocaine (Emla cream), can be placed under an occlusive bandage on an area of skin for sixty minutes before a painful skin-piercing procedure, resulting in decreased pain when the skin is pierced. Pain may present itself through a chronic dry mouth after radiation treatments. New products to help this condition (called *xerostomia*) include gels and artificial saliva in spray form. The medicine pilocarpine also can increase saliva production.

Fatigue Control

Fatigue, now recognized as a significant quality-of-life concern, is experienced by more than 70 percent of cancer patients. Yet many treatments are now possible. They must be based on understanding the various intervening causative factors. These include anemia, anorexia with wasting (often a result of cancer cells producing or stimulating the production of large amounts of the immune system products called *cytokines*), radiotherapy (a side effect for 60 percent of people two or three weeks after radiotherapy has started is fatigue), immunotherapy, chronically disrupted sleep, chemotherapy, major surgery, chronic pain, anxiety, depression, loneliness, or a combination of all of these. Treatments include teaching relaxation response and other stress management techniques, learning special forms of breathing, stretching, and exercise for improved sleep; learning how to pace yourself, modifying expectations and self-image, all for improved coping. Medications such as the steroid megestrol acetate, which produces improved appetite, weight gain, and improved sense of well-being, can help; appropriate use of stimulants (Ritalin, dexedrine) can improve energy; judicious use of acupuncture and massage can improve relaxation; proper use of antidepressants, antianxiety agents, and sleep medicines can improve overall sense of well-being.

Bone Marrow and Stem Cell Transplants

Transplants of liver, kidneys, and other organs as part of the treatment for cancer are relatively uncommon at this time. Bone marrow transplantation, while controversial, is increasing rapidly in its use for patients with aplastic anemia, recurrent breast cancer, leukemia, and lymphoma. Bone marrow transplantation allows very aggressive use of chemotherapy with or without radiation. When treatments two to five times greater than normal are delivered, the therapeutic goal is to kill all diseased cells in the body. Such aggressive treatment also destroys the patient's immune system and blood cells (red cells and platelets). Rescue of the patient is accomplished through bone marrow transplantation.

Ideally, if a transplant is recommended, you will be able to use either your own pretreatment bone marrow (called an *autologous transplant*) or baby blood cells, called *stem cells*, harvested from your blood (peripheral stem-cell rescue). *Allogeneic transplants* come from donors. They can be lifesaving but obviously present a greater risk for serious side effects and failure than using cells from your own body. This treatment presents a major challenge to you, your family, the medical team, and health insurance payment systems. Costs run $100,000 or more. There is a risk to your life, although in experienced hands we no longer see the 25 percent mortality rates of several years ago. Death as a result of complications such as overwhelming infection from the procedure ranges from 3 to 15 percent of all patients. Although clear questions exist concerning its real benefit for patients such as those with metastatic breast cancer—does it improve quality of life and lengthen survival?—a slowly increasing number of state governments are requiring that bone marrow transplants be covered by insurance plans operating within those states. Among those states are Massachusetts, New Hampshire, Vermont, and Virginia.

Immunotherapies and Vaccines

The idea that our immune systems help destroy cancer cells, now a documented fact, drives much of the research in immunotherapies. The intent is to find ways to improve the aggressiveness and effectiveness of the immune system in its ability to identify and then destroy unwanted cells without injuring the rest of the body. Because many cancer cell lines, once established in the body, are no longer recognized as undesirable cells by the immune system, this reality adds significantly to the challenge of creating successful immunotherapies.

Vaccines are a long-established method to increase immune system activity against infectious illnesses. They hold great appeal in the fight against the cancers. The effectiveness and appeal of vaccines, once developed, relies greatly on the fact—mentioned much earlier in this book—that the immune system, just like our brain, has a memory, often lifelong. Hence the wish for a way to prevent cancer is encouraged by the idea that vaccines might be developed.

Can vaccines be made against tumor cells with the same positive results that we find with vaccines against infectious agents? Increasing efforts are being made to do just that, despite the fact that no identified tumor-associated antigen is truly specific only to that tumor. Until recently the best results reported for vaccines having therapeutic effectiveness tended to be in the 25 percent range for cancer regression; this resulted in vaccines being discredited in the 1970s as not sufficiently effective to be considered a part of cancer treatment.

Despite a past filled with many disappointments, there are in the late 1990s various new, intriguing successes. One example involves the clinical experiments of Larry Kwak, M.D., and his colleagues at the National Cancer Institute. For selected individuals with myeloma his research group took protein molecules from a patient's cancer cells and then injected them into a healthy sibling to stimulate an immune reaction to the new, foreign-to-the-sibling's-body proteins. This reaction stimulated the healthy sibling's immune cells to vigorously attack any substance or cell having those proteins on its surface. Then bone marrow cells from the now-sensitized healthy sibling were infused into the sibling ill with myeloma. The hope was that these infused, sensitized cells would multiply and attack the myeloma cells. That is indeed what happened, producing a significant regression in the cancer. Experimental therapies using various forms of vaccines are currently being carried out with malignant melanoma and lymphoma.

Most likely, the greatest hope for vaccines lies in prevention (see the next section). For those cancers that have a viral infection as a necessary initial step in the cascade of events resulting in the development of cancer cells, vaccines can be created. We have already done this for hepatomas (one common form of liver cancer) with a vaccine against hepatitis B. The future is promising for the eventual development of vaccines against the Epstein-Barr virus

(Burkitt's lymphoma, nasopharyngeal carcinoma, B-cell lymphomas), papilloma virus (anogenital cancers in women and men), and human T-cell lymphotropic viruses (adult T-cell leukemia and adult T-cell lymphoma).

Immunotherapies distinct from vaccines currently rely on the use of cytokines and monoclonal antibodies used alone or in combination with chemotherapy and radiotherapy. Cytokines are natural regulating substances produced by immune system cells; that is, their purpose is either to increase or to decrease the expansion and the activity of that system. More than fifty cytokines have been identified. Only a very few, such as tumor necrosis factor (TNF), have the capacity to directly kill tumor cells. Cytokines already have a place in cancer treatment. They can be used in combination with cytotoxic drugs. When the cytokine called *interferon (IFN)* is used with the well-known antimetabolite called *5-fluorouracil (5-FU),* it has been shown to reverse the resistance of tumors to 5-FU. When TNF is combined with the antimetabolites Adriamycin, doxorubicin, and etoposide, the destruction of tumor cell DNA is enhanced. When the cytokine called *interferon alpha* is added to a four-drug regimen (doxorubicin, cyclophosphamide, vincristine, and prednisone), the result is a significant prolongation of remission time and overall survival for patients with non-Hodgkin's lymphoma.

Certain cytokines can interact with one another, producing an enhancement of tumor-killing activity. This effect has shown some promise in the treatment of one form of melanoma and in fibrosarcomas. Cytokines naturally can enhance the antitumor aggressiveness of certain cells in the immune system. Learning to build on this capacity is the object of current study. In one example, the cytokine interleukin-2 (IL-2) has been shown to dramatically increase the activity of the type of lymphocyte called *natural killer cells* (*NK cells*), transforming them into cells designated lymphokine-activated killer cells (LAK cells). Finally, some cytokines when infused in large amounts have direct therapeutic effects. One of the most successful examples involves the three-times-per-week subcutaneous injection of interferon alpha-2a in combination with vinblastine chemotherapy. This combination has increased survival for some patients with renal cancer.

Another treatment approach involves stimulating the immune system by infusing an immune system product called *monoclonal antibodies*. A monoclonal antibody is a special protein made by cells that have been challenged by a specific invading substance; that protein either inactivates the unwanted foreign substance or tags it as undesirable in a fashion that attracts immune system cells to it, which then have the ability to eliminate the substance from the body or render it harmless. Monoclonal antibodies can be made in the laboratory and mass produced from a single family of sensitized-to-the-unwanted-substance cells. One such substance called Panorex (Centocor/Glaxo companies) was approved in Germany in 1994 for the treatment of cancer. Other designer antibodies exist. They include anti-B-1 (also called anti-CD20), which, when given intravenously, significantly helps patients who have a CD20-positive form of B-cell lymphoma (50 percent remission, some long term), and IDEC-C2B8 monoclonal antibody, which in relapsed non-Hodgkin's lymphoma patients proves less toxic than chemotherapy and more active in killing tumor cells.

Today these designer antibodies help in the treatment of a very few cancers. They cure no cancers at this point. We still have much to learn.

Gene Therapy

The range and speed of change, of improvement, in all dimensions of cancer makes your hopeful expectations reasonable. Gene therapy, so much in the news beginning in 1995, although no longer science fiction, presents a setup for false hope over the short term. It may, however, take its place in the therapeutics of some cancers during the next five years.

What does all this mean to you? You want hope for yourself, your family, and others who love you. You want to see a diminishment, even an elimination, of fearful expectations and other forms of suffering. All you wish for may soon come to pass.

Genetics

Your awareness that some cancers—colon, breast, ovarian—are associated with genetic alterations that are conveyed from one generation to another has been stimulated through television, radio, newspapers, and magazines over the last five years. Does knowledge of genetics lead to new ways of treating, maybe even beating cancer? Can we learn how to attack or get rid of bad genes or of substances produced by defective genes that influence normal cells to become cancers?

In answering this, let us first review some basic information. All cells have genetic material within them. That genetic material, DNA and RNA, directs all cell function and proliferation. Small instructional segments on the strands of DNA in cells are called *genes*. *Oncogenes* refer to normal genes that become renegades in their function through spontaneously arising mutations, starting the cells on the path to becoming cancer cells by giving them a signal to divide permanently. Oncogene mutations are not inherited. *Protooncogenes* refer to mutated genes that directly turn normal cells into cancer cells. These are the genes associated with early-onset breast and ovarian cancer (BRCA 1) and multiple endocrine neoplasia (MEN-2A and -2B). *Tumor suppressor genes* refer to genes that are expert copy-editors or quality assurance officers, checking out the accuracy of protein-manufacturing instructions that come from the gene libraries on the chromosomes (DNA strands) in our cells; they also produce proteins that are involved with the regulation of cell proliferation. When tumor suppressor genes suffer from a mutation, they lose their normal function—that is, they lose their quality assurance authority, producing deviant protein that allows, through a complex process, excessively successful cell replication. The cells never stop replicating—the cells become immortalized, no longer team players in a balanced system. Such immortalized cells are cancer cells. Mutations in tumor suppressor genes can persist in a family, resulting in that family having a higher risk for certain cancers. Nothing is simple in biologic systems. Probably for cancers to exist, multiple mutations in both classes of genes must occur. (For example, we now know that at least six genetic alterations are required to get small-cell lung cancer started.) Now, how does knowledge of these things help us with new treatments for cancer?

Research studies have now documented that mutations in the p53 and p16 tumor suppressor genes are found in about 50 percent of all known cancers. Mutations in p53 are found in 100 percent of small-cell lung cancers, 70 percent of colon cancers, and 30 to 50 percent of breast cancers. This leads to the idea that one treatment strategy possibly could be to develop techniques for introducing normal tumor suppressor genes into cancer cells. Theoretically, they would take control by generating normal proteins, returning cancer cells to normal behavior: slowing down replication and making the cells mortal again. Techniques have been developed using harmless retroviruses that readily infect cells. These tiny viruses act as carriers into tumor cells for nonmutant (healthy) genes. Other approaches using viral vectors involve introducing cytokine genes that would "jazz up" the production of interleukin-2 (IL-2) by cancer cells. These theoretically would turn cancer cell function toward their own destruction because the increased IL-2 secretion would summon more natural killer cells, enhancing their killing activity by converting them into LAK cells, which would in turn attack and destroy the cancer cells. As we learn more about genetics, the possibilities for introducing genes to interfere specifically with the functioning, growth, and replications of cancer cells continues to expand.

Early Identification and Prevention

Diagnosis and Screening

Developments in the early diagnosis of cancer continue to evolve very rapidly. There is an increasing use of serum tumor markers, specific proteins produced by rapidly growing tumor cells, that can be identified through blood tests. The presence of these tumor-specific proteins can be quantified through blood tests, giving an approximate idea of how active a cancer in a particular individual might be.

Tests in wide use include CEA (carcinoembryonic antigen) and PSA (prostate specific antigen). Both CA 125 and CA 125-II have been approved for serum identification of ovarian cancer. Other serum tests in existence include CA 72-4 for gastrointestinal cancer, CA 15-3 for breast cancer, and CYFRA 21-1 for lung cancer.

In certain parts of the world viral titers in the blood help with the early detection of cancer. For example, 5 percent of adults in China with high Epstein-Barr virus titers (IgA) have been found when screened by flexible endoscopy to have evidence of very early nasopharyngeal cancer despite appearing to be entirely healthy. Early identification and treament can produce cures.

Physics contributes in many ways. One of the newer approaches to early diagnosis and screening involves single photon emission computed tomograph (SPECT scanning). This technology allows for multidimensional images based on radioactive emissions from injected trace compounds that cancer cells ingest and use much faster than normal cells. As a result in SPECT scan images any tumor cells make themselves known by glowing in contrast to normal tissue in the pictures.

Remember that genes are segments of DNA that carry the instructions for cells concerning how to manufacture proteins. Proteins play many different roles in both the function (chemical reactions) and structure of cells. These DNA segments can be transferred and replicated as part of cell replication. They can also be transferred by infecting bacteria and viruses. Today we have learned to both isolate and selectively transmit genes. The result is an explosively developing knowledge about genes and how they are associated with cells becoming cancerous.

This knowledge about genes in turn leads to an increasing ability, called *genetic diagnostics*, to predict risk. Its positive dimension is that individuals at risk for various cancers can be recognized and offered aggressive prevention and surveillance programs with the intent of identifying developing cancer for treatment as early as possible. The following table illustrates some of the current cancer-related genes for whose protein products diagnostic tests have been or are being developed.

Genetics Diagnostics

Genes	Cancer
BRCA 1; BRCA 2; BRCA 3	Breast
MSH2; MLH 1	Colon
MSH2	Uterine and ovarian
MEN-2A and B; RET	Endocrine
p 16	Melanoma
p 53	Li-Fraumeni syndrome
CD-19	Leukemia/lymphoma

Prevention

During the twentieth century we have tracked down and demonstrated the effects on living organisms of all kinds of environmental toxins, from coal tar and its derivatives to DDT, Agent Orange, radioactive elements, and the PCBs. These toxins produce changes in the genetic mechanisms as well as in the energy-producing systems of cells. They result in sterility, deviant growth, or cell death. The deviant growth often presents itself in the form of some kind of cancer.

One recent example is occurring in children exposed through the Chernobyl accident to neck radiation. As they get older they are at higher risk for developing thyroid cancer.

Over the last ten years you may have read of scientific studies that have demonstrated more clearly the effects of background radiation, especially radon through the basements of homes and exposure to sunlight. Ultraviolet radiation's accumulated effects contribute to various forms of skin cancer, the squamous and basal cell carcinomas, and especially the melanomas. Radon's effects contribute over time to the develoment of lung cancer. Thus, prevention efforts focus more and more on not only cleaning up identified environmental toxins but also promotion of information and education so as to change people's behavior as one of the most powerful ways to decrease the incidence of cancer in the population. Education must continue to be directed aggressively toward eliminating the smoking and chewing of tobacco as well as encouraging people to use—behavioral change is required here—proper ventilation of basement air in high-radon areas, sun block, protective clothing, gloves, and masks for specific kinds of chemical exposure.

Industrial medicine and medical technology focus their efforts on the work environment. As a result, exposure to diagnostic x-rays (used in medicine, manufacturing, and security) is continuously monitored, controlled, and reduced. In clinical care the amount of radiation a patient receives from a CAT scan today is often much less than from a single chest x-ray thirty years ago. Asbestos has been significantly reduced as a presence in the workplace and schools. Therefore, the risk of developing the fatal lung tumors called *mesotheliomas* is reduced significantly. PCBs are used less frequently and when used handled more carefully. Electomagnetic radiation is also more carefully monitored today than in the past, even though its importance in the development of cancers remains questionable.

The monitoring of our food and water supply increases in importance. Few people are aware of the unsung heroes of the Food and Drug Administration and Department of Agriculture laboratories. Their constant vigilance protects us from acute poisoning, bacterial and viral diseases, and powerful cancer-producing toxins. For example, inspection of the peanut crops is essential for the identification of peanuts infected by a particular fungus whose by-product, aflatoxin, is an almost certain death sentence because of its powerful liver cancer–inducing capabilities.

Increasing knowledge of viral infections, including how our bodies and their cells respond to such intruders, opens totally new avenues to the prevention of cancer. A major recent example involves the viral infections that produce the chronic inflammation of the liver called *hepatitis B.* This chronic inflammation is associated with the eventual development of a cancer originating in the liver called *hepatoma.* Infection is readily transmitted from infected to noninfected people by blood, saliva, and fecal contamination. A vaccine, given in three stages over six months, has been developed that protects people from getting hepatitis B. This vaccine is a major step forward in the protection of all who work in high-risk situations. It provides encouragement to development of other antiviral vaccines for conditions such as hepatitis C, the Epstein-Barr virus, the human immunodeficiency virus (HIV) and its associated cancers of Kaposi's sarcoma as well as the non-Hodgkin's lymphomas.

Finally, never ignore the increasing information about nutrition and its relationship to the development of the cancers. Although challenged as being little more than a rallying flag for consumers ten years ago, it is now quite clear that the normal American diet—high in saturated fat and low in fiber—is associated with a clear increase in the prevalence of cancers of the colon, stomach, and urinary systems. Over the next five to ten years we will understand a great deal more about the cancer prevention importance of the antioxidant vitamins, vegetables (especially the cruciferous vegetables—cabbage and broccoli being two examples), or foods such as grapes that carry enzymes (special proteins) that seem to neutralize cancer-causing (cell-damaging) chemicals, as well as the preventive and healing roles of trace minerals, particularly selenium, molybdenum, zinc, and manganese.

In summary, I ask you to be aware of known risk factors to the development of the cancers. Use that awareness to engage in personal prevention where possible and to support community prevention activites directed toward minimizing or eliminating those risk factors. The following table summarizes the known cancer risk factors.

You see, your expectations are reasonable. You want hope for yourself, your family, and others who love you. You want to see fearful expectations and other forms of suffering diminished, even eliminated. All that you wish for may come to pass.

Some Cancer Risk Factors

Diet

High saturated fats and low fiber

Toxic Agents and Minerals	**Infectious Agents**	**Forms of Radiation**
Aflatoxin	Hepatitis B	ultraviolet
Asbestos	Hepatitis C	x-rays
Coal tar	Epstein-Barr virus	gamma rays
Coal tar derivatives		
Tobacco smoke		
PCBS		
Benzene		
Radium		
Uranium		
Chromium		

Appendix E: Cancer Centers, Books, and Other Resources

I'VE DIVIDED THIS APPENDIX into five sections. The first lists and describes cancer centers of excellence in the United States; the second, national government information sources; the third, nonprofit organizations dedicated to cancer patients; the fourth, Internet sources for those with computers available; and finally, some selected recommended publications.

Some of the information may be useful today; some months from now, but sooner or later these sources can inform you, save you time, and serve you well. Information enhances your participation in your treatment. As always, I wish you my best as you work to find the best solutions for your health and well-being.

U.S. Cancer Centers

Where do you go when you wish to seek a second or third opinion? For cancers currently treated in standardized ways such as early breast cancer, uncomplicated leukemia, or early Hodgkin's disease, second opinions with a board-certified oncologist in your community may be sufficient. For other cancers, using the PDQ system (see page 303), you may choose to seek that opinion from one of the cancer treatment centers that follow. Sometimes your physical presence is not needed; history, pathology slides, and study reports will do.

As I write this, certain centers stand out in terms of their expertise for specific cancers. I have selected them in collaboration with colleagues who I believe are objective and knowledgeable. But things change; institutions and their experts change. Reassurance comes from knowing that all cancer centers share information with one another. Furthermore, any oncologist in this country can, if so motivated, consult with any other oncologist, no matter where located.

For the sarcomas:

Dana Farber Cancer Institute, Boston, Massachusetts

Memorial Sloan-Kettering Cancer Center, New York, New York

For advanced Hodgkin's Disease:

Yale Comprehensive Cancer Center, New Haven, Connecticut

Stanford University School of Medicine, Palo Alto, California

For the lymphomas:

Memorial Sloan-Kettering Cancer Center, New York, New York

Dana Farber Cancer Institute, Boston, Massachusetts

M. D. Anderson Cancer Center, Houston, Texas

For brain tumors:

M. D. Anderson Cancer Center, Houston, Texas

Johns Hopkins Oncology Center, Baltimore, Maryland
University of California Hospital, San Francisco, California
New York University School of Medicine, New York City

For recurrent breast cancers:
Lombardi Cancer Research Center, Georgetown University, Washington, D.C.
Johns Hopkins Oncology Center, Baltimore, Maryland
Dana Farber Cancer Institute, Boston, Massachusetts
M. D. Anderson Cancer Center, Houston, Texas

For advanced prostate cancer:
Johns Hopkins Oncology Center, Baltimore, Maryland
Memorial Sloan-Kettering Cancer Center, New York, New York

For many of the cancers of children:
St. Jude Children's Research Hospital, Memphis, Tennessee
Texas Children's Cancer Center, Houston, Texas
Children's Hospital of Los Angeles, California
Dana Farber Cancer Institute, Boston, Massachusetts
Pediatric Oncology Branch, NCI, NIH, Bethesda, Maryland

For bone marrow transplants:
Fred Hutchinson Cancer Research Center, University of Washington, Seattle, Washington

Federally Funded Cancer Centers

(Source: Cancer Information Service, National Cancer Institute)

With the passage of the National Cancer Act in 1971, Congress formally recognized the need for an interdisciplinary approach to cancer treatment, research, and education. The resulting Cancer Centers Program now supports a total of fifty-four centers of four types: twenty-six comprehensive cancer centers, twelve basic science cancer centers, fifteen clinical cancer centers, and one consortium cancer center. All centers have developed special areas of expertise.

Comprehensive Cancer Centers

Alabama

University of Alabama at Birmingham Comprehensive Cancer Center
Birmingham, Alabama
Albert F. LoBuglio, M.D., Director
Janis T. Zeanah, Communications Coordinator
(205) 934-0282 or fax 934-1608

Arizona

Arizona Cancer Center, University of Arizona
Tucson, Arizona
Sydney E. Salmon, M.D., Director
Laurie Young, Director of Communications and Outreach
(520) 626-4413 or fax 626-2284

California

Jonsson Comprehensive Cancer Center, UCLA
Los Angeles, California
Rodney H. Withers, M.D., Interim Director
Anne M. Gadelha, Administrative Assistant
(310) 206-2805 or fax 206-9058

Kenneth Norris Jr. Comprehensive Cancer Center
University of Southern California
Los Angeles, California
Peter A. Jones, Ph.D., Director

Gail Sidney, Director of Public Relations
(213) 342-2653 or fax 342-1623

Connecticut

Yale Comprehensive Cancer Center
New Haven, Connecticut
Vincent T. DeVita, Jr., M.D., Director
Marion Morra, Associate Director of Cancer Information Services and Community Outreach
(203) 865-2665 or (203) 785-4095 or fax 785-4116

District of Columbia

Lombardi Cancer Research Center, Georgetown University Medical Center
Washington, D.C.
Marc E. Lippman, M.D., Director
Virginia Brown, Director of Marketing
(202) 784-3102 or fax 687-5718

Florida

Sylvester Comprehensive Cancer Center, University of Miami Medical School
Miami, Florida
Azorides R. Morales, M.D., Director
Cherie Rogers, Director of Public Relations
(305) 548-4302 or fax 548-4303

Maryland

Johns Hopkins Oncology Center
Baltimore, Maryland
Martin D. Abeloff, M.D., Director
Kate Ruddon, Public Relations Director
(410) 955-1287 or fax 614-2611

Massachusetts

Dana Farber Cancer Institute
Boston, Massachusetts
Christopher Walsh, Ph.D., Director
Regina D. Vild, Director of Public Affairs
(617) 632-4090 or fax 632-4050

Michigan

University of Michigan Comprehensive Cancer Center
Ann Arbor, Michigan
Max S. Wicha, M.D., Director
Maria McKinney, Director of Marketing and Public Relations
(313) 936-9584 or fax 936-9582

Michigan Cancer Foundation
Detroit, Michigan
Richard J. Santen, M.D., Interim Director
Joseph Michaels, Director of Public Relations
(313) 833-0710 or fax 993-7165

New Hampshire

Norris Cotton Cancer Center
Hanover, New Hampshire
R. Robert Greenberg, M.D.
Sherry Calkins, Director of Public Affairs
(603) 650-4284 or fax 650-2008

New York

Memorial Sloan-Kettering Cancer Center
New York, New York
Paul A. Marks, M.D., President
Avice Meehan, Vice President of Public Affairs
(212) 639-3573 or fax 639-3576

Roswell Park Cancer Institute
Buffalo, New York
Thomas B. Tomasi, M.D., Ph.D., Director
Joyce Buchnowski, Director of Public Affairs
(716) 845-8182 or fax 845-3575

Kaplan Comprehensive Cancer Center
New York University
New York, New York
Vittorio Defendi, M.D., Director
David Sachs, Acting Director of Public Affairs
(212) 263-5488 or fax 263-8425

North Carolina

Duke Comprehensive Cancer Center
Durham, North Carolina
J. Dirk Inglehart, M.D., Acting Director
David B. Rice, Acting Director of Communications
(919) 684-5731 or fax 684-5797

Lineberger Comprehensive Cancer Center
University of North Carolina
Chapel Hill, North Carolina
Joseph S. Pagano, M.D., Director
Dianne G. Shaw, Director of Communications
(919) 966-3036 or fax 966-3015

Cancer Center of Wake Forest University, Bowman Gray School of Medicine
Winston-Salem, North Carolina
Frank M. Torti, M.D., Director
Bob Conn, Science Writer
(910) 716-4977 or fax 716-6841

Ohio

Ohio State University Comprehensive Cancer Center
Columbus, Ohio
David E. Schuller, M.D., Director
Earle Holland, Associate Executive Director
(614) 292-8384 or fax 292-0154

Pennsylvania

Fox Chase Cancer Center
Philadelphia, Pennsylvania
Robert C. Young, M.D., President
Eric T. Rosenthal, Director of Public Affairs
(215) 728-2799 or fax 728-2594

University of Pennsylvania Cancer Center
Philadelphia, Pennsylvania
John H. Glick, M.D., Director
Lisa Feinstein, Manager Media Relations
(215) 349-8368 or fax 349-8312

Pittsburgh Cancer Institute
Pittsburgh, Pennsylvania
Ronald B. Herberman, M.D., Director
Lauren Ward, Medical News Bureau
(412) 624-2607 or fax 624-3184

Texas

The University of Texas M.D. Anderson Cancer Center
Houston, Texas
Charles A. LeMaistre, M.D., President
Stephen C. Stuyck, Associate Vice President of Public Affairs
(713) 792-3030 or fax 794-4418

Vermont

Vermont Cancer Center, University of Vermont
Burlington, Vermont

Richard J. Albertini, M.D., Ph.D., Director
Joan MacKenzie, Communications Director
(802) 656-4414 or fax 656-8788

Washington

Fred Hutchinson Cancer Research Center
Seattle, Washington
Robert W. Day, M.D., Ph.D., President and Director
Susan Edmonds, Media Relations Manager
(206) 667-2896 or fax 667-7005

Wisconsin

University of Wisconsin Comprehensive Cancer Center
Madison, Wisconsin
Paul P. Carbone, M.D., Director
Scott Hainzinger, Communications Coordinator
(608) 263-3223 or fax 263-6394

Clinical Cancer Centers

California

City of Hope National Medical Center
Beckman Research Institute
Duarte, California
John Kovach, M.D., Director
Laurel DiBrog, Manager, Marketing/News Services
(800) 888-5323 or fax (818) 301-8462

University of California–San Diego Cancer Center
San Diego, California
William M. Hryniuk, M.D., Director
Nancy Stringer, Assistant Director to Health Sciences Communications
(619) 543-6163 or fax 543-5423

University of California, Irvine Cancer Center
Orange, California
Frank L. Meyskens, Jr., M.D., Director
Susan Solomon, UCI Marketing and Public Relations
(714) 456-5496 or fax 456-8872

Colorado

University of Colorado Cancer Center
Denver, Colorado
Paul A. Bunn, Jr., M.D., Director
Connie Printz, Director of Cancer Communications
(303) 270-3021 or fax 270-3304

Illinois

University of Chicago Cancer Research Center
Chicago, Illinois
Richard L. Schilsky, M.D., Director
John Easton, Director of Media Affairs
(312) 702-6241 or fax 702-3171

Lurie Cancer Center
Northwestern University
Chicago, Illinois
Steven Rosen, M.D., Director
Deborah Barron, Public Affairs Director
(312) 871-9176 or fax 908-6346

Minnesota

Mayo Clinical Cancer Center
Rochester, Minnesota
Franklin G. Prendergast, M.D., Ph.D., Interim Director
Kay M. Thiemann, Communications Coordinator
(507) 284-3413 or fax 284-1803

New York

Albert Einstein College of Medicine
Bronx, New York
Mathew D. Scharff, M.D., Director
Art Oshins, Media Relations Manager
(718) 430-3101 or fax 824-7280

Columbia-Presbyterian Cancer Center
New York, New York
I. Bernard Weinstein, M.D., Director
Marie DePeri, Program Coordinator
(212) 305-9330 or fax 305-7846

University of Rochester Cancer Center
Rochester, New York
Richard F. Borch, M.D., Ph.D., Director
Susan Hyde Scholl, Assistant Director for Communications
(716) 273-4143 or fax 273-1042

Ohio

Ireland Cancer Center
Case Western Reserve University
Cleveland, Ohio
Nathan A. Berger, M.D., Director
Joanne R. Gambosi, R.N., M.A., Director of Cancer Information and Service and Community Outreach
(216) 844-5432 or fax 844-7832

Tennessee

St. Jude Children's Research Hospital
Arthur W. Nienhuis, M.D., Director
Jerry Chipman, Director of Public Relations
(901) 522-0306 or fax 525-2720

Texas

San Antonio Cancer Institute
San Antonio, Texas
Charles A. Coltman, Jr., M.D., Director
Jeannie Frieden, Director of Public Affairs
(210) 616-5580 or fax 692-9823

Utah

Utah Regional Cancer Center, University of Utah Health Sciences Center
Salt Lake City, Utah
Raymond W. White, Ph.D., Director
Heidi Smith, Administrative Manager
(801) 581-4048 or fax 585-5763

Virginia

Massey Cancer Center, Medical College of Virginia
Richmond, Virginia
I. David Goldman, M.D., Director
J. Sheppard Haw, III, Public Relations Specialist
(804) 828-1451 or fax 828-8453

Basic Science Cancer Centers

California

La Jolla Cancer Research Foundation
La Jolla, California
Erkki Ruoslahti, M.D., President and Scientific Director
Terry Gach, Vice President, Resource Programs
(619) 455-6480 or fax 455-0181

Armand Hammer Center for Cancer Biology
The Salk Institute
San Diego, California
Walter Echkhart, Ph.D., Director

Anita Weld, Public Relations Director
(619) 453-4100 ext. 1225 or fax 453-3015

Indiana

Purdue Cancer Center, Purdue University
West Lafayette, Indiana
William M. Baird, Ph.D., Director and Media Contact
(317) 494-9129 or fax 494-9193

Maine

The Jackson Laboratory
Bar Harbor, Maine
Kenneth Paigen, Ph.D., Director
Jeffre Witherly, Manager Public Information
(207) 288-3371 or fax 288-4152

Massachusetts

Center for Cancer Research, Massachusetts Institute of Technology
Cambridge, Massachusetts
Richard O. Hynes, Ph.D., Director and Media Contact
(617) 253-6422 or fax 253-8357

Nebraska

Eppley Institute, University of Nebraska Medical Center
Omaha, Nebraska
Raymond R. Ruddon, Jr., M.D., Ph.D., Director
Terrill Chappell, Editor/Coordinator
(402) 559-4232 or fax 559-4651

New York

Cold Spring Harbor Laboratory
Cold Spring Harbor, New York
Bruce W. Stillman, Ph.D., Director
Susan Cooper, Public Affairs Director
(516) 367-8455 or fax 367-8496

American Health Foundation
New York, New York
Ernst L. Wynder, M.D., President & Medical Director
Clara Horn, Executive Assistant to the President
(212) 551-2520 or fax 689-2339

Pennsylvania

Wistar Institute Cancer Center
Philadelphia, Pennsylvania
Giovanni Rovera, M.D., Director
Heidi Boorstein, Director of Public Affairs
(215) 898-3927 or fax 898-3715

Fels Research Institute, Temple University School of Medicine
Philadelphia, Pennsylvania
E. Premkumar Reddy, Ph.D., Director
Robert Villier, Director of Public Relations
(215) 707-4839 or fax 707-8012

Virginia

University of Virginia Cancer Center
Charlottesville, Virginia
Charles E. Meyers, Jr., M.D., Director
Anne Oplinger, Director, Health Sciences Center News Office
(804) 924-5679 or fax 982-4378

Wisconsin

McArdle Laboratory for Cancer Research, University of Wisconsin
Madison, Wisconsin
Norman R. Drinkwater, Ph.D., Director
Betty Sheehan, Public Affairs Director
(608) 262-8651 or fax 262-2824

Consortium Cancer Center

California

Drew-Meharry-Morehouse Consortium Cancer Center
Charles R. Drew University
Los Angeles, California
Louis J. Bernard, M.D., Director
Cynthia Dupree, Senior Analyst
(313) 754-2961 or fax 755-1036

Selected National Government Resources

National Cancer Institute (NCI)
Cancer Information Service
Building 31, Room 10A16
9000 Rockville Pike
Bethesda, MD 20892
1-800-4-CANCER (for Cancer Information Service)
(301) 402-5874 CANCERFAX
e-mail: cancernet@icicc.nci.nih.gov

Provides a nationwide telephone service paid for with your tax dollars for cancer patients and their families and friends, the public, and health care professionals. Answers questions and sends booklets about cancer. CANCERFAX provides treatment guidelines, with current data on prognosis, relevant staging and histologic classifications, news, and announcements of important cancer-related issues. Call CANCERFAX from your fax machine. Both CANCERFAX and 1-800-4-CANCER can instruct you on how to access the Physician Data Query (PDQ) system. That system provides information about the latest treatment approaches for all known cancers, where these treatments are being conducted, research studies, and studies looking for participants.

Agency for Health Care Policy & Research (AHCPR)
Clearinghouse
PO Box 8547
Silver Spring, MD 20907
1-800-358-8285

National Library of Medicine
1-800-638-8480

Office of Alternative Medicine
National Institutes of Health
Building 31, Room 5B-37
Bethesda, MD 20892
(301) 402-2466 or fax 402-4741

Selected Private Nonprofit Organizations

There are hundreds of advocacy, information, and support organizations in the United States. For reasons of space, this must be only a partial list. I mean no slight to other legitimate organizations I have left out. I have included the organizations that serve the largest numbers of cancer patients and their families.

American Brain Tumor Association
2720 River Rd., Suite 146
Des Plaines, IL 60018
1-800-886-2282 or fax (847) 827-9918
e-mail: ABTA@aol.com

Offers free services including publications about brain tumors, support group lists, referral information, and a pen pal program.

American Cancer Society (ACS)
1599 Clifton Rd., N.E.
Atlanta, GA 30329
1-800-ACS-2345 or (404) 320-3333
CanSurmount
I Can Cope
International Association of Laryngectomees
Look Good, Feel Better
Man to Man
Reach to Recovery
Road to Recovery

Dedicated to eliminating cancer as a major health problem through research, education, advocacy, and service.

American Institute for Cancer Research (AICR)
1759 R St., N.W.
Washington, DC 20009
1-800-843-8114 (nutrition hotline)
(202) 328-7744 (in Washington, DC)
(202) 328-7226 (fax)
Internet address: AICR.ORG

The AICR is the only major national cancer organization that supports research and provides public education exclusively in the area of diet, nutrition, and cancer.

Biofeedback Certification Institute of America
10200 West 44th Ave., Suite 304
Wheatridge, CO 80033
(303) 420-2902

Burger King Cancer Caring Center
4117 Liberty Ave.
Pittsburgh, PA 15224
(412) 622-1212 or fax 622-1216

Dedicated to helping people diagnosed with cancer, their families, and their friends cope with the emotional impact of cancer.

Cancer Fund of America
2901 Breezewood Ln.
Knoxville, TN 37921
(615) 938-5281

On a nationwide basis, this organization provides financial assistance to cancer patients.

Candlelighters Childhood Cancer Foundation
7910 Woodmont Ave., Suite 460
Bethesda, MD 20814-3015
(301) 657-8401 or 1-800-366-2223 or fax (301) 718-2686
e-mail: 75717.3515@compuserve.com

Provides information, support, and advocacy to families of children with cancer, survivors of childhood cancer, and professionals who work with them.

Commonweal Cancer Health Program
PO Box 316
Bolinas, CA 94924
(415) 868-0970

Corporate Angel Network (CAN)
Westchester County Airport Building 1
White Plains, NY 10604
(914) 328-1313 or fax 328-3938

Helps cancer patients in stable condition find free flights to and from recognized cancer treatment centers, using empty seats on corporate aircraft flying on normal business.

Hospice Foundation of America
2001 S St., N.W., Suite 300
Washington, DC 20009
(202) 638-5419 or fax 638-5312
777 17th St., Suite 401
Miami, FL 33139
(305) 538-9272 or fax 538-0092

Hospice Foundation of America provides leadership in the development and application of hospice and its philosophy of care with the goal of enhancing the American health care system and the role of hospice within it. It offers a monthly newsletter, an annual bereavement teleconference, and assorted publications and videotapes.

International Cancer Alliance (ICA)
4853 Cordell Ave., Suite 11
Bethesda, MD 20816
1-800-ICARE-61

This organization works to link patients, physicians, and cancer researchers through conferences and published-information exchange.

Leukemia Society of America
600 Third Ave.
New York, NY 10016
1-800-955-4LSA (educational materials)
(212) 573-8484 (general information)
(212) 856-9686 (fax)

Dedicated to seeking the cause and eventual cure of leukemia and related cancers. Nationwide programs include research, patient aid, public and professional education. The society offers local family support group programs, free of charge, to patients, families, and friends.

Lymphoma Research Foundation of America, Inc.
2318 Prosser Ave.
Los Angeles, CA 90064
(310) 470-4912 or fax 470-8502
e-mail: LRFA@aol.com

A nonprofit organization that funds research grants for projects seeking to cure lymphoma and improve treatments. It also provides education and free support groups for patients and their families and a national "buddy system" linking patients.

Make Today Count
c/o Connie Zimmerman
Mid-America Cancer Center
1235 E. Cherokee
Springfield, MO 65804-2263
1-800-432-2273 or fax (417) 888-7426

A mutual support organization that brings together persons affected by a life-threatening illness so they may help each other.

National Alliance of Breast Cancer Organizations (NABCO)
9 E. 37th St., 10th Floor
New York, NY 10016
1-800-719-9154 or fax (212) 689-1213
e-mail: NABCOinfo@aol.com

Source of information on breast cancer. Advocates for legislative and regulatory concerns of breast cancer community.

National Bone Marrow Transplant Link (BMT Link)
29209 Northwestern Hwy., #624
Southfield, MI 48034
1-800-LINK-BMT (phone and fax)

Promotes public understanding and peer support for those affected by bone marrow transplantation.

National Brain Tumor Foundation
785 Market St., Suite 1600
San Francisco, CA 94103
1-800-934-CURE
(415) 284-0208 or fax 284-0209

Pursues two major goals: providing support and education for brain tumor patients and finding a cure.

National Breast Cancer Coalition

1707 L St., N.W., Suite 1060
Washington, DC 20036
(202) 296-7477 or fax 265-6854

A grassroots advocacy movement of more than three hundred member organizations and thousands of individuals working through a national action network, dedicated to the eradication of breast cancer through research, access, and influence.

National Coalition for Cancer Survivorship (NCCS)

1010 Wayne Ave., 5th Floor
Silver Spring, MD 20910
(301) 650-8868 or fax 565-9670

Exists to enhance the quality of life for cancer survivors and to promote an understanding of cancer survivorship.

National Council Against Health Fraud Resource Center

300 E. Pink Hill Rd.
Independence, MO 64057
(816) 228-4595 or (909) 824-4690 in California

A helpful organization dedicated to collecting and disseminating information on questionable treatments and organizations.

National Family Caregivers Association

9621 East Bexhill Dr.
Kensington, MD 20895
1-800-896-3650 or fax (301) 942-2302

Provides information, education, support, and validation to America's family caregivers, the general public, and policy makers.

National Hospice Organization (NHO)

1901 N. Moore St., Suite 901
Arlington, VA 22209
1-800-658-8898 or fax (703) 525-5762

Provides general information about hospice programs and offers referrals.

National Kidney Cancer Association
1234 Sherman Ave., Suite 200
Evanston, IL 60202
(847) 332-1051 or fax 328-4425, BBS 332-1052

Works to increase the survival of kidney cancer patients and improve their care by providing information, sponsoring research, and acting as an advocate on behalf of patients.

National Marrow Donor Program
3433 Broadway St., N.E., Suite 500
Minneapolis, MN 55413
1-800-MARROW-2 or fax (612) 627-5877

A congressionally authorized network that maintains a computerized data bank of available tissue-typed marrow donor volunteers nationwide.

National Patient Air Transport Hotline (NPATH)
PO Box 1940
Manassas, VA 22110
1-800-296-1217 or fax (703) 361-1792

Makes referrals to all known appropriate charitable, charitably assisted, and special patient discount commercial air transport services based on an evaluation of patient's needs.

Oley Foundation
214 Hun Memorial
Albany Medical Center A-23
Albany, NY 12208
1-800-776-OLEY or fax (518) 262-5528

Support for home parenteral and/or enteral nutrition therapy consumers and their families through a newsletter, conferences, meetings, outreach, and support activities.

R. A. Bloch Cancer Foundation, Inc.
The Cancer Hotline
4410 Main St.
Kansas City, MO 64111
(816) 932-8453 or fax 931-7486

Helps people diagnosed with cancer have the best possibility of beating it as easily as possible through informational resources, peer counseling, medical second opinions, and support groups.

Ronald McDonald House
Ronald McDonald House Charities
One Kroc Dr.
Oak Brook, IL 60521
(708) 575-7048 or fax 575-7488

Offers a refuge from the hospital, a "home away from home."

Support for People with Oral and Head and Neck Cancer, Inc. (SPOHNC)
PO Box 53
Locust Valley, NY 11560-0053
(516) 759-5333 (phone and fax)

Self-help program of support addressing the broad emotional, psychological, and humanistic needs of these cancer survivors, empowering each to take an active role in his or her recovery.

Susan G. Komen Breast Cancer Foundation
5005 LBJ Freeway, Suite 370
Dallas, TX 75244
1-800-IM AWARE or fax (214) 450-1710

A national volunteer organization working through local chapters and Race for the Cure events across the country, fighting to eradicate breast cancer by advancing research, education, screening, and treatment. The Helpline is answered by trained volunteers who provide information to callers with breast health or breast cancer concerns.

United Ostomy Association, Inc.
36 Executive Park, Suite 120
Irvine, CA 92714
1-800-826-0826 or (714) 660-8624 or fax 660-9262

Association of ostomy chapters dedicated to complete rehabilitation of all ostomates.

US TOO International, Inc.
930 North York Rd., Suite 50
Hinsdale, IL 60521-2993
1-800-808-7866 or (708) 323-1002 or fax 323-1003

Provides prostate cancer survivors and their families emotional and educational support through an international network of chapters.

Y-ME
National Breast Cancer Organization
212 W. Van Buren, 4th Floor
Chicago, IL 60607
1-800-221-2141 or 24-hour hotline (312) 986-8228
or fax 986-0020

Hotline counseling, educational programs, and self-help meetings for breast cancer patients, their families, and friends.

Y-ME Men's Support Line
M–F 9 A.M.–5 P.M. CST

Men can call the Y-ME 800 number and request to speak to a male counselor. The counselor most closely matched in experience to the caller will return the call within twenty-four hours.

Selected Internet Sites

It is possible to drown in the information available on the Internet. Many of the sources are of unknown quality and reliability. What follows are the current best and reliable sources of cancer information.

1. CancerNet: National Cancer Institute

   http://www.icic.nci.nih.gov

   Basically, this gives PDQ system information. It is updated every month.

2. OncoLink: Univ. of Pennsylvania Cancer Center

   http://oncolink.upenn.edu

   Cancer information from causes to costs to treatment.

3. American Cancer Society

   http://www.cancer.org

In addition to the preceding, there are disease-specific Web sites, mailing lists, discussion groups, and chat lines. New in 1997 is the Healthfinder Web site maintained by the U.S. government (DHHS) offering links to more than 300 federal Web sites and 500 Web sites of state and local governments, universities, and not-for-profit organizations.

http://www.healthfinder.gov

Selected Recommended Publications

1. Cancer Information Service of the National Cancer Institute. Call 1-800-4-CANCER and ask to be sent the current publications list. Most of the publications are filled with useful information reviewed by experts and written by professionals. These publications are free and for the most part equal or exceed the quality of anything you can buy in a bookstore.
2. American Cancer Society. Your local chapter will often have the publication list and some publications. The society's booklets on sexuality and cancer are excellent.
3. National Coalition for Cancer Survivorship. The coalition has excellent booklets on employment rights, health insurance, and talking with your doctor.
4. *Coping* magazine. A bimonthly publication that is the only nationally distributed consumer magazine for people whose lives have been touched by cancer.
   PO Box 682268
   Franklin, TN 37068-2268
   (615) 790-2400 or fax 794-0179
   e-mail: Copingmag@aol.com

Selected Recommended Books

There are many good books on various aspects of cancer. I have avoided the temptation to try to make this as complete as possible. I believe that the books listed both as references and as of general interest will provide you new information and perspectives. They each have some valuable lessons to share with you on cancer and coping.

Reference Books

Complete Drug Reference. Yonkers, New York: Consumer Reports Books, 1997.

Goleman, Daniel, and Joel Gurin, eds. *Mind/Body Medicine: How to Use Your Mind for Better Health.* Yonkers, New York: Consumer Reports Books, 1993.

Grossinger, Richard. *Planet Medicine: Origins* and *Planet Medicine: Modalities.* Berkeley, California: North Atlantic Books, 1995.

Hoffman, Barbara, ed. *A Cancer Survivor's Alamanac: Charting Your Journey.* Minneapolis: Chronimed Publishing (an NCCS publication), 1996.

Lerner, Michael. *Choices in Healing: Integrating the Best of Conventional and Complementary Approaches to Cancer.* Cambridge, Massachusetts: MIT Press, 1994.

NIH publication no. 94-066. *Alternative Medicine: Expanding Medical Horizons.* Washington, D.C.: U. S. Government Printing Office, 1994.

Other Books

Benson, Herbert, and E. Stuart. *The Wellness Book: The Comprehensive Guide to Maintaining Health and Treating Stress-Related Illness.* Secaucus, New Jersey: Carol Publishing Group, 1992.

Eisenberg, David, with Thomas Lee Wright. *Encounters with Qi: Exploring Chinese Medicine.* New York/London: Penguin Books, 1987.

Love, Susan M., with Karen Lindsey. *Dr. Susan Love's Breast Book.* Second Edition. Massachusetts/California/New York: Addison-Wesley, 1995.

Price, Reynolds. *A Whole New Life.* New York: Simon and Schuster, 1994.

Seuss, Dr. *You're Only Old Once! A Book for Obsolete Children.* New York: Random House, 1986.

Spiegel, David. *Living Beyond Limits: A Scientific Mind-Body Approach to Facing Life-Threatening Illness.* New York: Fawcett, 1994.

Spingarn, Natalie Davis. *Hanging in There: Living Well on Borrowed Time.* New York: Stein and Day, 1982.

Index